Mapping of Atrial Tachycardias Post-Atrial Fibrillation Ablation

Editors

ASHOK J. SHAH
MICHEL HAISSAGUERRE
SHINSUKE MIYAZAKI

CARDIAC ELECTROPHYSIOLOGY CLINICS

www.cardiacEP.theclinics.com

Consulting Editors
RANJAN K. THAKUR
ANDREA NATALE

June 2013 • Volume 5 • Number 2

ELSEVIER

1600 John F. Kennedy Boulevard • Suite 1800 • Philadelphia, Pennsylvania, 19103-2899

http://www.theclinics.com

CARDIAC ELECTROPHYSIOLOGY CLINICS Volume 5, Number 2
June 2013 ISSN 1877-9182, ISBN-13: 978-1-4557-7068-7

Editor: Barbara Cohen-Kligerman
Developmental Editor: Teia Stone

Cardiac Electrophysiology Clinics (ISSN 1877-9182) is published quarterly by Elsevier Inc., 360 Park Avenue South, New York, NY 10010-1710. Months of issue are March, June, September, and December. Subscription prices are $191.00 per year for US individuals, $277.00 per year for US institutions, $100.00 per year for US students and residents, $214.00 per year for Canadian individuals, $309.00 per year for Canadian institutions, $273.00 per year for international individuals, $331.00 per year for international institutions and $143.00 per year for Canadian and foreign students/residents. To receive student/resident rate, orders must be accompanied by name of affiliated institution, date of term, and the signature of program/residency coordinator on institution letterhead. Orders will be billed at individual rate until proof of status is received. Foreign air speed delivery is included in all Clinics subscription prices. All prices are subject to change without notice. **POSTMASTER:** Send address changes to Cardiac Electrophysiology Clinics, Elsevier Health Sciences Division, Subscription Customer Service, 3251 Riverport Lane, Maryland Heights, MO 63043. **Customer Service: 1-800-654-2452 (US and Canada). From outside of the US and Canada, call 314-477-8871. Fax: 314-447-8029. E-mail: JournalsCustomerService-usa@elsevier.com (for print support); JournalsOnlineSupport-usa@elsevier.com (for online support).**

Reprints. For copies of 100 or more of articles in this publication, please contact the Commercial Reprints Department, Elsevier Inc., 360 Park Avenue South, New York, NY 10010-1710. Tel.: 212-633-3812; Fax: 212-462-1935; E-mail: reprints@elsevier.com.

Printed and bound by CPI Group (UK) Ltd, Croydon, CR0 4YY

Transferred to digital print 2013

Contributors

CONSULTING EDITORS

RANJAN K. THAKUR, MD, MPH, MBA, FHRS
Professor of Medicine and Director, Arrhythmia
Service, Thoracic and Cardiovascular Institute,
Sparrow Health System, Michigan State
University, Lansing, Michigan

ANDREA NATALE, MD, FACC, FHRS
Executive Medical Director, Texas Cardiac
Arrhythmia Institute, St David's Medical
Center, Austin, Texas; Consulting Professor,
Division of Cardiology, Stanford University,
Palo Alto, California; Adjunct Professor of
Medicine, Heart and Vascular Center, Case
Western Reserve University, Cleveland, Ohio;
Director, Interventional Electrophysiology,
Scripps Clinic, San Diego, California; Senior
Clinical Director, EP Services, California Pacific
Medical Center, San Francisco, California

EDITORS

ASHOK J. SHAH, MD
Departments of Electrophysiology, Cardiac
Arrhythmias, and Rhythmologie, Hôpital
Cardiologique du Haut-Lévêque, Université
Victor Segalen Bordeaux II, Bordeaux-Pessac,
France

MICHEL HAISSAGUERRE, MD
Department of Rhythmologie, Hôpital
Cardiologique du Haut-Lévêque, Université
Victor Segalen Bordeaux II, Bordeaux-Pessac,
France

SHINSUKE MIYAZAKI, MD
Department of Rhythmologie, Hôpital
Cardiologique du Haut-Lévêque, Université
Victor Segalen Bordeaux II, Bordeaux-Pessac,
France

AUTHORS

THOMAS ARENTZ, MD
Arrhythmia Department, Universitäts-
Herzzentrum Freiburg – Bad Krozingen,
Bad Krozingen, Germany

MICHEL HAISSAGUERRE, MD
Department of Rhythmologie, Hôpital
Cardiologique du Haut-Lévêque, Université
Victor Segalen Bordeaux II, Bordeaux-Pessac,
France

MATTHEW DALY, MD
Department of Rhythmologie, Hôpital
Cardiologique du Haut-Lévêque, Université
Victor Segalen Bordeaux II, Bordeaux-Pessac,
France

MELEZE HOCINI, MD
Department of Electrophysiology, Hôpital
Cardiologique du Haut-Lévêque, Université
Victor Segalen Bordeaux II, Bordeaux-Pessac,
France

AMIR S. JADIDI, MD
Arrhythmia Department, Universitäts-Herzzentrum Freiburg – Bad Krozingen, Bad Krozingen, Germany; Departments of Electrophysiology, Arrhythmia, and Rhythmologie, Hôpital Cardiologique du Haut-Lévêque, Université Victor Segalen Bordeaux II, Bordeaux-Pessac, France

PIERRE JAIS, MD
Department of Rhythmologie, Hôpital Cardiologique du Haut-Lévêque, Université Victor Segalen Bordeaux II, Bordeaux-Pessac, France

SEBASTIEN KNECHT, MD
Department of Rhythmologie, Hôpital Cardiologique du Haut-Lévêque, Université Victor Segalen Bordeaux II, Bordeaux-Pessac, France

YUKI KOMATSU, MD
Department of Rhythmologie, Hôpital Cardiologique du Haut-Lévêque, Université Victor Segalen Bordeaux II, Bordeaux-Pessac, France

HEIKO LEHRMANN, MD
Arrhythmia Department, Universitäts-Herzzentrum Freiburg – Bad Krozingen, Bad Krozingen, Germany

XING-PENG LIU, MD
Department of Cardiology, Beijing Chao-Yang Hospital, Capital Medical University, Beijing, China; Department of Rhythmologie, Hôpital Cardiologique du Haut-Lévêque, Université Victor Segalen Bordeaux II, Bordeaux-Pessac, France

SEIICHIRO MATSUO, MD
Department of Rhythmologie, Hôpital Cardiologique du Haut-Lévêque, Université Victor Segalen Bordeaux II, Bordeaux-Pessac, France

SHINSUKE MIYAZAKI, MD
Department of Rhythmologie, Hôpital Cardiologique du Haut-Lévêque, Université Victor Segalen Bordeaux II, Bordeaux-Pessac, France

CHAN-IL PARK, MD
Arrhythmia Department, Universitäts-Herzzentrum Freiburg – Bad Krozingen, Bad Krozingen, Germany

PATRIZIO PASCALE, MD
Department of Cardiology, Centre Hospitalier Universitaire Vaudois et Université de Lausanne, Lausanne, Switzerland; Departments of Electrophysiology, Cardiac Arrhythmias, and Rhythmologie, Hôpital Cardiologique du Haut-Lévêque, Université Victor Segalen Bordeaux II, Bordeaux-Pessac, France

MICHALA PEDERSEN, MD
Department of Electrophysiology, Hôpital Cardiologique du Haut-Lévêque, Université Victor Segalen Bordeaux II, Bordeaux-Pessac, France

LAURENT ROTEN, MD
Department of Cardiology, Inselspital, Bern University Hospital, University of Bern, Bern, Switzerland; Department of Cardiac Arrhythmias, Hôpital Cardiologique du Haut-Lévêque, Université Victor Segalen Bordeaux II, Bordeaux-Pessac, France

FREDERIC SACHER, MD
Department of Electrophysiology, Hôpital Cardiologique du Haut-Lévêque, Université Victor Segalen Bordeaux II, Bordeaux-Pessac, France

ASHOK J. SHAH, MD
Departments of Electrophysiology, Cardiac Arrhythmias, and Rhythmologie, Hôpital Cardiologique du Haut-Lévêque, Université Victor Segalen Bordeaux II, Bordeaux-Pessac, France

REINHOLD WEBER, MD
Arrhythmia Department, Universitäts-Herzzentrum Freiburg – Bad Krozingen, Bad Krozingen, Germany

XU ZHOU, MD
Department of Cardiology, Beijing Chao-Yang Hospital, Capital Medical University, Beijing, China

Contents

facilitate the diagnostic process. In the first step, irregularity in cycle length (or recurrent spontaneous onset/offset) is diagnostic of focal AT. The second step has been devised to help the operator confirm or rule out macroreentrant AT, because there are limited possibilities and mapping of a few points on the path (circuit) is adequate to reach the diagnosis. After macroreentry has been ruled out, focal AT is the only possibility; its localization requires mapping of the entire chamber.

Diagnosis of Focal-Source Atrial Tachycardia: Localized Reentry and Focal Atrial Tachycardia

Michala Pedersen, Ashok J. Shah, Patrizio Pascale, and Meleze Hocini

Focal-source atrial tachycardias (ATs) are common following atrial fibrillation abla-tion. They can be hard to map, but with due patience and perseverance, the source of earliest activation can usually be located. It is very useful to first rule out a macro reentrant tachycardia, and following this, start homing in on the source. Mapping with a multi-electrode may help pinpoint the earliest site and can often allow dem-onstration of activity spanning most of the tachycardia cycle length. Once entrain-ment has confirmed the source of the AT, the target can be ablated.

Typical Examples of Focal-Source Atrial Tachycardia

Michala Pedersen, Amir S. Jadidi, Frederic Sacher, and Meleze Hocini

In this article examples of the mapping of focal-source atrial tachycardias are pre-sented. The aim is to underpin the strategies for mapping these atrial tachycardias as described in the other articles in this issue. Each case contains many individual examples of maneuvers. It is worthwhile spending time on each figure and under-standing the mapping technique used.

Misleading Features of Activation and Entrainment Mapping

Ashok J. Shah, Shinsuke Miyazaki, Xing-Peng Liu, Yuki Komatsu, Patrizio Pascale, and Pierre Jais

The following atypical features of activation and entrainment mapping may be encountered during the diagnostic mapping of atrial tachycardias. (1) Unusual dis-parate activations of the coronary sinus and the contiguous left atrium, which can be deciphered by magnifying the recordings on the coronary sinus bipoles. (2) After entrainment of tachycardia, the return cycle length (postpacing interval) may seem shorter than the tachycardia cycle length. (3) Despite the site lying close to the reen-trant circuit, the return cycle length (postpacing interval) after entrainment may be much longer than 30 ms because of altered conduction in the local area.

Exotic Atrial Tachycardias

Ashok J. Shah, Shinsuke Miyazaki, Sebastien Knecht, Seiichiro Matsuo, Matthew Daly, Yuki Komatsu, Patrizio Pascale, Laurent Roten, and Meleze Hocini

Atrial tachycardias (ATs) arising after atrial fibrillation ablation are mechanistically macroreentrant or focal-source (including localized reentry) ATs. They are usually more than 1 and occur in succession as ablation subtly converts one AT to another. This article discusses rare forms of AT such as double ATs with coexisting similar or different mechanisms, AT coexisting with sinus rhythm, and a focal-source AT mimicking macroreentry. These unusual cases underscore the importance of careful mapping and observation during the invasive procedure and show how ablation modifies the atrial substrate harboring the ATs.

Serial Atrial Tachycardias: Importance of Subtle Changes

Shinsuke Miyazaki, Ashok J. Shah, and Pierre Jais

A series of successive atrial tachycardias may be encountered after atrial fibrillation ablation. The conversion of atrial tachycardia may be obvious or subtle. A subtle change of electrogram sequence, cycle length, or surface P wave, or no apparent

CARDIAC ELECTROPHYSIOLOGY CLINICS

Foreword
"Needle in a Haystack"

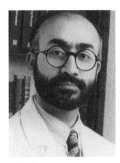 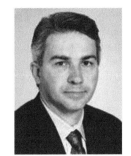

Ranjan K. Thakur, MD, MPH, MBA, FHRS   Andrea Natale, MD, FACC, FHRS
Consulting Editors

Catheter ablation for atrial fibrillation (AF) has been one of the most exciting developments in cardiac electrophysiology. The initial observation that AF may originate from focal electrical firing, often within the pulmonary veins, launched the AF ablation era. But ablation inside the culprit vein was fraught with complications and various "isolation" and containment techniques were championed by various laboratories around the world to prevent electrical communication between the source and the remainder of the atrium. Unfortunately, these approaches also have their problems, namely, postablation organized atrial tachyarrhythmias.

These organized atrial tachyarrhythmias can be focal, localized-reentrant, or macro-reentrant. More than one arrhythmia or arrhythmia mechanism may coexist, and they may be seen in more than one-third of the patients after an index AF ablation procedure, especially when AF had been persistent or longstanding persistent. It is possible that the incidence may be even higher since only the symptomatic arrhythmias come to light. A detailed delineation of the mechanism and the circuit is required in order to target ablation lesions effectively, but these arrhythmias can be difficult to map and ablate, and varying success rates have been reported. Chasing these arrhythmias, intellectually, is one of the most difficult challenges we face, not unlike finding "a needle in a haystack."

The electrophysiology laboratory in Bordeaux, France, headed by Dr Michel Haissaguerre, described the pulmonary vein triggers for AF and has been at the forefront in the "fight against AF." While they use many of the newer advanced mapping technologies to map and ablate these complex arrhythmias, they rely heavily on the traditional, labor-intensive, hardcore electrophysiologic techniques to elucidate and map these difficult arrhythmias. Such a rigorous approach is required and skipping these techniques to resort to colorful 3-dimensional maps may mislead and result in low success rates.

The editors of this issue of the *Cardiac Electrophysiology Clinics*, Drs Shah, Haissaguerre, and Miyazaki, and their contributors (representing the first- and third-generation Bordeaux electrophysiologists) have illustrated many of these electrogram-based, "conventional" principles of localizing these arrhythmias. The topics include discussion ranging from the basic principles of conventional mapping, optimizing signal acquisition, differentiating right from left atrial tachycardias, to developing a practical mapping algorithm, misleading features of activation and entrainment mapping, and illustrated examples of a variety of tachycardias. While the emphasis is clearly on conventional techniques, they also discuss the role of 3-dimensional mapping for atrial tachycardias and an emerging technology, body surface mapping, to study these arrhythmias noninvasively. Most of the figures were created specifically for this audience so as to illustrate as clearly as possible the rigor involved in studying these arrhythmias. The editors and contributors have devoted incredible effort to convey

Card Electrophysiol Clin 5 (2013) xi–xii
http://dx.doi.org/10.1016/j.ccep.2013.03.001
1877-9182/13/$ – see front matter © 2013 Published by Elsevier Inc.

cardiacEP.theclinics.com

these teaching points. The reader is well advised to avail the teachable moment and study these figures in detail, for indeed each "picture is worth a thousand words."

Ranjan K. Thakur, MD, MPH, MBA, FHRS
Sparrow Thoracic and Cardiovascular Institute
Michigan State University
1200 East Michigan Avenue; Suite 580
Lansing, MI 48912, USA

Andrea Natale, MD, FACC, FHRS
Texas Cardiac Arrhythmia Institute
Center for Atrial Fibrillation at
St. David's Medical Center
1015 East 32nd Street; Suite 516
Austin, TX 78705, USA

E-mail addresses:
thakur@msu.edu (R.K. Thakur)
andrea.natale@stdavids.com (A. Natale)

Preface

Mapping of Atrial Tachycardias Post Atrial Fibrillation Ablation

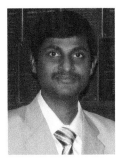

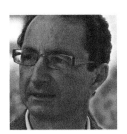

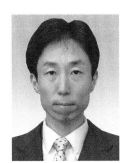

Ashok J. Shah, MD   Michel Haissaguerre, MD   Shinsuke Miyazaki, MD

Editors

Atrial tachycardias arising in the context of catheter ablation of atrial fibrillation (AF) require a systematic approach for successful ablation and long-lasting remission. These arrhythmias are frequently (but not only) encountered during the ablation of persistent AF when fibrillatory activity transforms into a more organized and uniform pattern of atrial tachycardia/flutter. They can also be the presenting clinical problem after one or more previous ablations for AF, which, together with remodeling of the atria, may provide a favorable substrate for the development of sustained atrial tachycardia. In either form, these arrhythmias are unique. They are usually more than one in number such that the road to sinus rhythm often marches through multiple forms of tachycardia (macro-reentry, localized reentry, or true focal point tachycardia). They manifest in rapid succession as ablation converts one form into another. They can be very fast to very slow. They are very often incessant, resistant to rate- and rhythm-control, and leave the patients in unbearable symptoms necessitating early ablation therapy. These arrhythmias require a patient and a methodical diagnostic approach followed by ablation at the optimal sites because random ablation can not only become proarrhythmic but also hamper appropriate diagnosis, subsequently.

Because we consider that it is important to spend time studying the ongoing arrhythmia using electrogram-based mapping techniques and ascertain the diagnosis before pushing the radiofrequency paddle, we endeavor to elucidate the principles of mapping atrial tachycardias arising post-AF ablation in an illustrated manner, including their obvious as well as subtle features. As we hope to present a practical approach for mapping post-AF ablation atrial tachycardias, this issue of *Cardiac Electrophysiology Clinics* has been written in the style of a manual more than as a reference text. In addition to the conventional approach, it includes 2 articles describing the pertinent roles of the advanced invasive and the recent noninvasive system in 3-dimensional atrial tachycardia mapping. It also includes electrogram recordings of several typical and atypical atrial tachycardias, which can be encountered in the clinical laboratory. The key points are summarized at the beginning of each article to facilitate understanding its contents. It is our sincere wish that this issue of *Cardiac Electrophysiology Clinics* will become a valuable part of every electrophysiology laboratory that is involved in AF ablation.

Last, but not the least, we would like to thank Professor Pierre Jais, whose deductive atrial tachycardia-diagnostic approach forms the basis

Card Electrophysiol Clin 5 (2013) xiii–xiv
http://dx.doi.org/10.1016/j.ccep.2013.02.003
1877-9182/13/$ – see front matter © 2013 Published by Elsevier Inc.

of the electrogram-based tachycardia mapping method described in this issue.

Ashok J. Shah, MD
Hôpital Haut Lévêque
33604 Bordeaux-Pessac, France

Michel Haissaguerre, MD
Hôpital Cardiologique du Haut Lévêque
Avenue de Magellan
33604 Pessac Cedex, France

Shinsuke Miyazaki, MD
Hôpital Haut Lévêque
Avenue de Magellan
33604 Bordeaux-Pessac
France

E-mail addresses:
drashahep@gmail.com (A.J. Shah)
michel.haissaguerre@chu-bordeaux.fr
(M. Haissaguerre)
mmshinsuke@gmail.com (S. Miyazaki)

Optimizing Signal Acquisition and Recording in an Electrophysiology Laboratory

Amir S. Jadidi, MD[a,b,*], Heiko Lehrmann, MD[a],
Reinhold Weber, MD[a], Chan-Il Park, MD[a],
Thomas Arentz, MD[a]

KEYWORDS

- Electrocardiography • Electrogram • Filtering • Amplitude • Fragmentation • Noise • Artifact
- Atrial and ventricular tachycardia

KEY POINTS

- Optimization of surface and intracardiac electrocardiogram (ECG) signal quality is a prerequisite for successful mapping of cardiac arrhythmia in the electrophysiology laboratory.
- Recommendations on filtering and amplification techniques for both surface and intracardiac ECGs assure diagnostic-quality ECGs, essential for the identification of arrhythmia sources and critical slow conduction sites within scarred myocardium.

INTRODUCTION

The correct diagnosis of arrhythmia is based on successful mapping in the electrophysiology laboratory, which depends on a high-quality display of both surface electrocardiogram (ECG) and intracardiac electrogram (EGM). This article discusses the optimal settings for acquisition of high-quality surface ECG and bipolar intracardiac recordings. Typical examples of noise (extrinsic) and artifacts (intrinsic) on surface ECG and intracardiac recordings are demonstrated.

SURFACE ECG

Recommended Settings for Diagnostic ECG Quality

Diagnostic ECG quality necessitates recording of the frequency spectrum starting at 0.05 Hz and reaching up to at least 100 Hz in adults, 150 Hz in adolescents, and 250 Hz in infants.[1–5] Reduction of this frequency spectrum by addition of notch/noise filters (50/60 Hz notch filters) attenuates high-frequency components within or after the P-QRS complex (**Fig. 1**A–C). Similarly, a reduction of low-pass filtering (35 Hz instead of the recommended minimum of 100 Hz) reduces the high-frequency components in the P-QRS. These components are of special interest for a detailed P-wave analysis in patients with atrial tachycardia and the exact morphologic analysis of the premature ventricular contractions (PVCs)/ventricular tachycardia (VT), the identification of high-frequency fragmented P-QRS components (eg, Epsilon waves in arrhythmogenic right ventricular dysplasia), and determination of the P-QRS amplitude and duration, which depend on the display of all its components. To measure routine P-QRS durations and amplitudes accurately in adults, adolescents, and children, an upper-frequency cutoff of at least 150 Hz is required;

Conflicts of Interest: None.
Disclosures: None.
[a] Arrhythmia Department, Universitäts-Herzzentrum Freiburg – Bad Krozingen, Südring 15, 79180 Bad Krozingen, Germany; [b] Arrhythmia Department, Hôpital Cardiologique du Haut-Lévêque and the Université Victor Segalen Bordeaux II, Bordeaux, France
* Corresponding author. Department of Rhythmology, Universitäts-Herzzentrum Freiburg – Bad Krozingen, Südring 15, 79180 Bad Krozingen, Germany.
E-mail address: amir.s.jadidi@gmail.com

Card Electrophysiol Clin 5 (2013) 137–142
http://dx.doi.org/10.1016/j.ccep.2013.01.005
1877-9182/13/$ – see front matter © 2013 Elsevier Inc. All rights reserved.

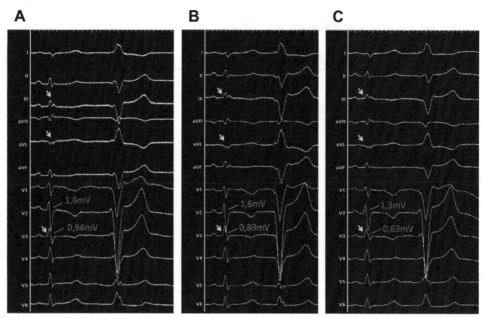

Fig. 1. *A:* 0.05–250 Hz without notch filter at 50 mm/sec speed and 1 mV/cm. *B:* 0.05–100 Hz without notch filter at 50 mm/sec speed and 1 mV/cm. *C:* 0.05–100 Hz with 50 Hz notch filter at 50 mm/sec speed and 1mV/cm. If the low-pass filter is reduced from 100 to 50 Hz, high-frequency components within or after the QRS complex are attenuated or may completely disappear. (*A, B*) There is little change in P-wave and QRS morphology of sinus beat and premature ventricular contraction when a notch filter is not added. However, addition of a 50-Hz notch filter (*C*) leads to an important reduction of the high-frequency components within the P wave and the QRS complex (*yellow arrows*). In addition, a significant reduction in the QRS voltages is noted.

an upper-frequency cutoff of 250 Hz is more appropriate for infants.[1,3–5]

Fig. 1 demonstrates loss of signal information within the QRS complexes in a patient with symptomatic PVC. **Fig. 1**A shows tracings with a complete frequency spectrum (0.05–250 Hz), and **Fig. 1**B demonstrates only slight differences in the P-wave and QRS patterns with filter range of 0.05 to 100 Hz and without the addition of a 50-Hz notch filter. However, adding a notch filter (50 Hz) is associated with significant reduction in ECG signal information (see **Fig. 1**C). Of note, significant ST elevations may be observed with a modified high-pass filter (HPF) setting at 0.1 Hz or higher. HPF settings have to be set at 0.05 Hz to prevent artificial ST elevations in surface ECG leads suggestive of ischemia, pericarditis, or mimicking of ECG patterns of Brugada syndrome.[1,2,6]

The voltage amplification of the 12-lead ECG is adapted to the underlying arrhythmia. The ECG amplitude may be enhanced to 0.2 mV/cm in the case of atrial tachycardia, to allow clear visualization of P-wave morphology and its earliest onset (**Fig. 3**).

Artifacts on Surface ECG

The 3 limb leads (I, II, III) on the 12-lead surface ECG use the voltage differences between the 2 respective electrodes to determine the direction of the electrical bipole within each extremity lead. The Goldberger leads (aVL, aVF, aVR) and Wilson precordial leads (V1–V6) use a common reference electrode to determine electrical voltage difference between the reference and the respective lead. The Wilson precordial leads act as "unipolar" electrodes: electrical forces directed toward each precordial electrode result in positive deflections and fleeing forces in negative deflections. To achieve the unipolar-like detection mode in the precordial leads, electrical voltages are measured with reference to a high-resistance reference (consisting of a simultaneous connection to the right-arm, left-arm, and left-leg electrodes with addition of a high resistance), the so-called Wilson central terminal. Therefore, artifacts concerning all precordial leads simultaneously are related to insufficient connection of extremity electrode(s) (right-arm, left-arm, or leg electrodes) to the patient's skin.

The connection to the right-leg electrode is important for further stabilization and noise reduction of the 12-lead ECG. A bad electrode-skin connection of the right-leg electrode introduces significant artifacts on the surface ECG. Disconnection of the right-leg electrode at baseline (**Fig. 2**A) and during atrial pacing (**Fig. 2**B) from the lateral right atrium catheter and is related with noise on

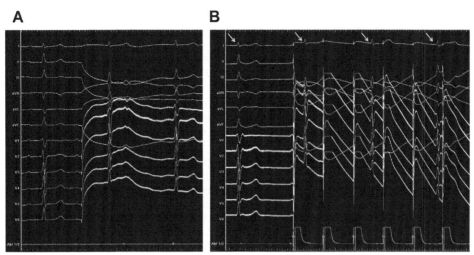

Fig. 2. (*A, B*) The connection to the right-leg electrode is important for stabilization and noise reduction of the 12-lead ECG. A bad electrode-skin connection of the right-leg electrode introduces important artifacts on the surface ECG. (*A*) The impact of disconnection of the right-leg electrode at baseline. (*B*) Disconnection of the right-leg electrode during pacing from lateral right atrium catheter, with important noise in the limb leads and baseline drift in all ECG leads. QRS complexes are barely seen (*yellow arrows*).

all surface ECG leads and a reduced cancellation of the pacing artifact from the surface ECG.[7]

INTRACARDIAC ECG RECORDING
Recommended Filter Settings for Intracardiac Bipolar ECG

Intracardiac electrograms (EGMs) require a different pass-band from surface ECG signals because of differences in frequency content and enhanced baseline drifting. Rejection of baseline drift is important, and a lower cutoff frequency of 30 Hz is widely used in bipolar recording mode. The authors recommend optimal filter settings for bipolar intracardiac EGMs of 30 to 250 Hz (the low-pass filter may alternatively be set higher, up to 500 Hz). Use of notch filters (50 or 60 Hz) or adaptive filters, which may reduce or remove

important local cardiac signals (see **Fig. 1**), should be avoided. A reduction of the low-pass filter to less than 250 Hz (eg, to 100 Hz) is not recommended, because of attenuation or cancellation of high-frequency electrogram contents that are essential for near-field EGMs from (1) pulmonary veins, (2) the electrical conduction system (His potential, bundle branches, and Purkinje system), and (3) scar-containing slow-conduction sites with fractionated high-frequency EGMs.

Recommended Voltage Amplification Settings for Intracardiac Bipolar ECG

For best detection and visualization of low-voltage fractionated EGMs at scar-related slow-conduction sites (diastolic potentials during reentrant tachycardias, see **Fig. 3**), the authors recommend

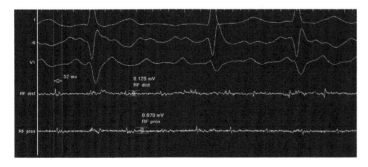

Fig. 3. Optimal amplification and filter settings for bipolar intracardiac electrograms (EGMs): 30 to 250 Hz or 30 to 500 Hz, without addition of any notch (50 or 60 Hz) filters or adaptive filters that may reduce or remove important local cardiac signals. In this case of scar-related localized reentry circuit at the left atrial roof, very low voltage (0.03–0.07 mV) fractionated EGMs were found at the critical isthmus of the atrial tachycardia. These potentials were mid-diastolic and preceded the earliest P wave by 52 milliseconds. Ablation at that site with the low-voltage diastolic potential terminated the atrial tachycardia. The voltage amplification of the 12-lead ECG is adapted to enable arrhythmia mapping. In this case, surface ECG amplitudes were enhanced to 0.2 mV/cm (at 100 mm/s) and RF electrograms were amplified at 0.4 mV/cm (at 100 mm/s speed) to allow clear visualization of P-wave morphology and its earliest onset.

a high level of EGM voltage amplification. The displayed voltage scale on the electrophysiology recording system screen should be adjusted as follows for the different catheter types. Radiofrequency (RF) catheter: 1 mV/40 mm to 1 mV/80 mm (corresponding to 0.125–0.25 mV/cm, depending on scar content); circumferential catheter (eg, Lasso [Biosense Webster, Diamond Bar, CA] for pulmonary vein mapping: 1 mV/20 mm to 1 mV/40 mm [corresponding to 0.5–0.25 mV/cm]). These crucial potentials may be as low as 0.03 mV (30 µV) within the dense scar regions, which may be essential components of a slowly conducting isthmus of a scar-related tachycardia (see **Fig. 3**).

EGM Saturation Versus Clipping

EGM saturation occurs at too high EGM amplification (gain or range settings on the amplifier). Reduction of the "gain" or adjustment of the displayed EGM "range" to a higher range eliminates signal cutting caused by saturation. By contrast, EGM clipping may be useful to display a smaller EGM (eg, His potential) at high amplification followed by a high-voltage EGM (eg, ventricular signal) that does not need to be visualized to its full extent (**Fig. 4**A, B). However, operators should be careful with catheter manipulation when the signals are clipped. High-voltage signals from thin-walled atrial regions (eg, right and left atrial appendages) can be truncated and not seen during EGM clipping. Therefore, catheter positioning should be performed with unclipped signals at usual amplification levels, so that even if the catheter inadvertently infiltrates thin-walled regions of cardiac chambers (atrial appendages or right ventricular outflow tract), the operator will be reminded about it by high-voltage EGMs from those regions.

Electrical Noise in the Electrophysiology Laboratory

The electrophysiology laboratory is a noisy electromagnetic environment, because of coexistence of a conglomerate of electrical equipment connected to the patient: ECG machine, RF-ablation generator, electroanatomic mapping and navigation system, intracardiac catheters and their connections to the amplifier system, external defibrillator, digital pulse oximeter, general anesthesia equipment such as ventilator, patient-warming ventilated cover, monitors/screens, and multiple main electricity suppliers of 50 Hz (220 V AC) or 60 Hz (120 V AC). External noise may also originate from mobile phones and wireless communication devices (headsets, monitors, computers, and so forth).

A very low noise level (<0.01 mV) allows identification of very low-voltage EGMs (from scarred areas as low as 0.03 mV, see **Fig. 3**), and the best strategy to achieve this is to avoid noise and artifacts by electromagnetic optimization of the electrophysiology laboratory. Interference between different pieces of the recording/amplifier system and other systems must be avoided. All patient connections must be electrically isolated (a mandatory safety requirement), leading to a reduction in the circulating currents at 50/60 Hz, which constitute the major source of interference in the electrophysiology laboratory. Electrical equipment should be plugged into wall sockets placed far apart from each other. Cables should be shortened to the minimum length required. Parallel course of ECG cables with RF-delivery cables and RF-catheter irrigation tubes should be avoided, to minimize noise on ECG (both surface and intracardiac) recordings. RF-catheter cable and power supply cables should not pass near to the amplifier pin-box (where intracardiac and surface ECGs are recorded by the amplifier system). Unused cables should be removed from the laboratory. The electrical power supply for the RF generator should be placed away from the generator, to avoid "contamination" of RF-catheter signal with 50/60 Hz noise. Further details on the technical background regarding ECG-signal processing and electrical noise in the electrophysiology laboratory have been published recently.[7]

Fig. 5B demonstrates an example of 50-Hz noise on an RF-ablation catheter that could be abolished by placing the RF generator further away from its electrical power supply. **Fig. 5**A shows a high-frequency noise (>120 Hz) caused by the catheter localization signal of the NavX (St Jude Medical, St Paul, MN) electroanatomic mapping system. On turning off the NavX catheter localization signal, the high-frequency noise disappears on both surface and intracardiac EGMs (EGMs on the left side in **Fig. 5**A). This high-frequency noise (EGMs on the right side in **Fig. 5**A) is often observed when the NavX system is used with the Bard (Lowell, MA) electrophysiology recording system. It most probably depends on the position and connection of surface ECG electrodes and RF-ablation reference patch relative to the position of NavX patches that transmit the localization signal. Future efforts and collaborations between developers of electroanatomic mapping systems and cardiac electrophysiology ECG amplifying/recording systems will, it is hoped, abolish or reduce such incompatibility issues between different electrophysiology systems, which are essential tools in today's electrophysiology laboratory.

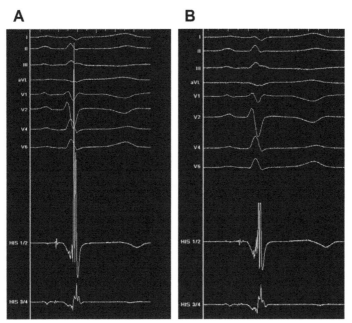

Fig. 4. EGM clipping. EGM clipping may be useful to display a smaller EGM (eg, His potential) at high amplification followed by a high-voltage EGM (eg, ventricular signal) that does not need to be visualized to its full extent. (*A*) Unclipped versus (*B*) clipped His-catheter signal.

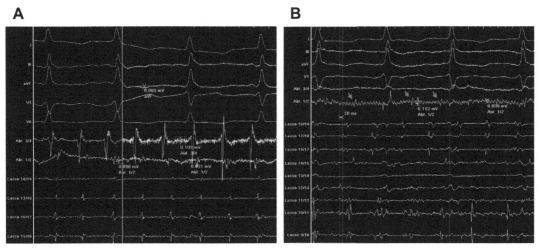

Fig. 5. (*A*) High-frequency noise (>120 Hz) caused by catheter localization signal of the NavX (St Jude Medical) electroanatomic mapping system (*right side of the blue vertical line*), which reached 0.1 mV amplitude on the proximal bipoles of the ablation catheter. When the localization signal is turned off (*left side of the blue vertical line*), the high-frequency noise disappears on both surface and intracardiac EGMs. (*B*) Noise of 50 Hz (cycle length 20 milliseconds) on RF-ablation catheter, which could be abolished by placing the RF generator further away from the electrical power supply. Note that the local atrial EGM voltage is 0.11 mV (*blue arrows*) and 50-Hz noise level is 0.06 mV. Electrogram amplifications at 100 mm/s speed were: Surface ECG 1 mV/20 mm (0.5 mV/cm); RF catheter 1 mV/40 mm (0.25 V/cm); Lasso catheter 1 mV/20 mm (0.5 mV/cm). The intracardiac EGM amplifications were enhanced up to 1 mV/80 mm (0.125 mV/cm) in the case of extensive scar and very low-voltage EGMs (0.03–0.2 mV).

REFERENCES

1. Kligfield P, Gettes L, Bailey J, et al. Recommendations for the standardization and interpretation of the electrocardiogram: part I: the electrocardiogram and its technology. A scientific statement from the American Heart Association Electrocardiography and Arrhythmias Committee, Council on Clinical Cardiology; the American College of Cardiology Foundation; and the Heart Rhythm Society endorsed by the International Society for Computerized Electrocardiology. J Am Coll Cardiol 2007;49:1109–27.
2. Berson AS, Pipberger HV. The low-frequency response of electrocardiographs, a frequent source of recording errors. Am Heart J 1966;71:779–89.
3. Zywietz C, Wagner GS, Scherlag BG, et al, editors. Sampling rate of ECGs in relation to measurement accuracy. Computerized interpretation of the electrocardiogram. New York: Engineering Foundation; 1986. p. 122–5.
4. Rijnbeek PR, Kors JA, Witsenburg M. Minimum bandwidth requirements for recording of pediatric electrocardiograms. Circulation 2001;104:3087–90.
5. Garson A Jr. Clinically significant differences between the "old" analog and the "new" digital electro-cardiograms. Am Heart J 1987;114:194–7.
6. Bragg-Remschel DA, Anderson CM, Winkle RA. Frequency response characteristics of ambulatory ECG monitoring systems and their implications for ST segment analysis. Am Heart J 1982;103:20–31.
7. Venkatachalam KL, Herbrandson JE, Asirvatham SJ. Signals and signal processing for the electrophysiologist part I: electrogram acquisition. Circ Arrhythm Electrophysiol 2011;4:965–73.

Basic Principles of Conventional Mapping

Xing-Peng Liu, MD[a,*], Xu Zhou, MD[a], Ashok J. Shah, MD[b]

KEYWORDS

- Atrial tachycardia • Atrial fibrillation • Entrainment • Activation mapping • Postpacing interval

KEY POINTS

- Fluoroscopy-based cardiac mapping techniques can be used for mapping atrial tachycardia after atrial fibrillation ablation.
- The local atrial activation time can be determined with intracardiac bipolar electrograms alone, providing a sharp local activation time in combination with unipolar electrograms, the morphology of which provides important information regarding wave genesis and propagation.
- Using conventional activation mapping and entrainment mapping techniques, most atrial tachycardia can be mapped accurately.

Currently, the management of atrial tachycardia (AT) after atrial fibrillation (AF) ablation is a major challenge for electrophysiologic (EP) practitioners, because this tachycardia is increasingly common, highly symptomatic, and refractory to antiarrhythmic drugs or multiple electrical cardioversions.[1] In fact, catheter ablation may be the only effective treatment available for most of these patients. Although 3-dimensional mapping, which may be helpful in interpreting the mechanisms of complex arrhythmias, is becoming popular in the EP community, conventional mapping techniques are still useful in mapping AT after AF ablation. Conventional mapping not only is an intrinsic part of any 3-dimensional mapping system but also provides more detailed information regarding the mechanisms of AT and suitable ablation targets. This article introduces basic principles of conventional mapping.

UNIPOLAR AND BIPOLAR SIGNALS

Intracardiac electrical signals recorded by catheter electrodes can provide 2 important types of electrogram: unipolar and bipolar. Although bipolar recordings may provide sufficient information for most of the mapping purposes in most clinical EP laboratories, simultaneous unipolar recording is also recommended because it can provide additional critical information, such as the more accurate local activation time and the direction of activation propagation.[2] Filtering is important for both unipolar and bipolar intracardiac electrograms. A typical high-pass filter setting for bipolar intracardiac electrograms is 30 to 50 Hz, and it preserves the high-frequency components and eliminates the low-frequency ones. Unipolar electrograms typically undergo high-pass filtering set at 0.05 Hz, which preserves the polarity and morphology of the signal. To eliminate noise at higher frequencies, low-pass filters are generally set to approximately 500 Hz for intracardiac signals because essentially no intracardiac signal components are of interest at higher than 300 Hz.[3]

The unipolar electrogram records the potential difference between a single electrode directly in contact with the heart (an "exploring" electrode, which is connected to the positive input of the

---

Conflict of Interest: None.
[a] Department of Cardiology, Beijing Chao-Yang Hospital, Capital Medical University, 8 Gong Ti Nan Road, Beijing 100020, China; [b] Hôpital Cardiologique du Haut-Lévêque, Bordeaux-Pessac 33604, France
* Corresponding author. Heart Center, Center for Atrial Fibrillation, Beijing Chao-Yang Hospital, Capital Medical University, 8 Gong Ti Nan Road, Chaoyang District, Beijing 100020, China.
E-mail address: xpliu71@gmail.com

Card Electrophysiol Clin 5 (2013) 143–152
http://dx.doi.org/10.1016/j.ccep.2013.01.004
1877-9182/13/$ – see front matter © 2013 Elsevier Inc. All rights reserved.

recording amplifier) and an "indifferent" electrode placed at a distance from the heart (such as in the inferior vena cava) or the Wilson central terminal. In fact, the unipolar recording is not truly unipolar because all recordings depend on voltage differences between 2 poles; the "unipolar" designation simply means that one of the poles is away from the heart.[4] The morphology of the unipolar electrogram plays an important role in determining the local activation propagation. In the case of activation propagation toward the mapping electrode, a positive deflection will be recorded (R waves). Accordingly, when the propagation is away from the mapping electrode, a negative deflection will be recorded (**Fig. 1**). If a recording electrode is just at the source of tachycardia, with all wavefronts spreading away from this site, a monophasic QS complex starting with a rapid downstroke will be recorded. **Fig. 2** presents an example of the QS pattern in the unipolar

electrogram for a patient with focal AT. The amplitude of the unipolar electrogram is proportional to the area of the dipole layer and the reciprocal value of the square of the distance between the dipole layer and the recording site. Thus, the unipolar electrogram records a combination of local (near-field) and remote (far-field) electrical events, with the contribution of far-field electrical events decreasing in proportion to the square of the distance from the mapping electrode. Additionally, unipolar recordings can provide a more precise measure of local activation. Normally, a unipolar signal has 3 time points: the point of maximal amplitude, the point of zero crossing, and the point of maximal negative change in potential with time (dV/dt). The maximum negative change in dV/dt is considered the best point reflecting the local activation time of myocardium directly beneath the electrode, because the maximal negative dV/dt corresponds to the maximum sodium channel conductance. Unipolar recordings have 2 major disadvantages. First, they have a poor signal-to-noise ratio and substantial far-field signals because of depolarization of tissue remote from the recording electrode. For patients with AT after AF ablation, this is especially true if aggressive ablation has been performed during the previous ablation procedures. Second, they are unable to record an undisturbed electrogram during or immediately after pacing.

The bipolar electrogram records the potential difference between 2 closely spaced electrodes in direct contact with the heart (see **Fig. 1**). Therefore, bipolar recordings can provide an improved signal-to-noise ratio, and high-frequency components that are more accurately observed. With 2 closely spaced electrodes (such as in the case of an ablation catheter), the timing of the far-field signal recorded on each of them is similar and is therefore subtracted out, making small local potentials easier to recognize. Local activation time is generally taken as the first rapid peak of the bipolar signal. In some situations, however, local activation time cannot be easily determined using the bipolar electrogram alone, such as in an area presenting double potentials because of previous ablation. In that case, the combination with unipolar electrograms is often helpful.

The major limitation of bipolar recordings lies in the lower directional sensitivity. For example, if the activation wavefront is parallel to the electrode pair, the bipolar spike will be of maximal amplitude, whereas if it is perpendicular to the electrode pair, the 2 electrodes will record the same waveform at the same time, and no spikes will be recorded. To acquire the more accurate local electrical activity, an electrode pair with a small (<10 mm) interelectrode distance is recommended.[2–5]

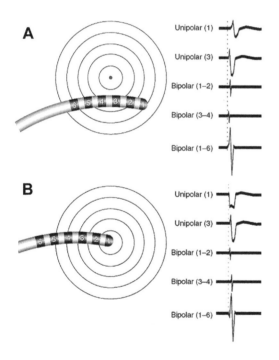

Fig. 1. Hypothetical recordings from a multipolar electrode catheter. (*A*) The electrodes are near a point source of activation (*dot in center of concentric rings*). Note the timing and shape of the resultant electrogram patterns based on the distance from the point source, unipolar or bipolar recording, and width of bipole. (*B*) The tip electrode (1) is at the point source of activation. Note differences in timing and shape of electrograms compared with A. (*Modified from* Issa ZF, Miller JM, Zipes DP. Clinical arrhythmology and electrophysiology: a companion to Braunwald's heart disease. Philadelphia: Saunders; 2009. p. 58; with permission.)

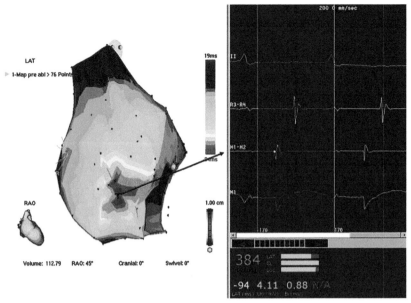

Fig. 2. Example of QS morphology in the unipolar recording at the site of earliest atrial activation in a patient with focal AT. The left panel shows 3-dimensional electroanatomic map of AT wherein the earliest atrial activation site is colored red. This site is located in the low lateral part of the right atrium and the activation time of the whole right atrium (113 ms) can be observed to be less than one-third of the AT cycle length (384 ms), suggesting the focal mechanism. The right panel shows the intracardiac recording from the site with the earliest atrial activation. From top to bottom are lead II, the proximal coronary sinus recoding (R3–R4), bipolar recording (M1–M2), and unipolar recording (M1) from the distal electrode of the mapping catheter. The unipolar electrogram has a QS pattern with a sharp downstroke, which is consistent with the electrogram morphology at the source of this focal AT.

ACTIVATION MAPPING

Activation mapping is the most important and commonly used mapping modality in the EP laboratory. For most ATs after AF ablation, the mechanism of AT, whether it be focal firing, localized reentry, or macroreentry, can be determined by locating the site of earliest atrial activation and tracing the atrial activation sequence during the AT.

Usually, activation mapping begins with assessment of atrial activation using catheters positioned at different routine sites in the high right atrium, coronary sinus (CS), and bundle of the His region. In initial arrhythmia evaluation, recording from these sites allows rough estimation of the site of interest. Although activation mapping simultaneously from as many atrial sites as possible can greatly enhance the precision, detail, and speed of identifying regions of interest, sequential atrial activation mapping using a roving catheter combined with a fixed CS mapping catheter is an alternative approach that is also effective in clarifying the mechanism of AT after AF ablation, and with noticeably lower cost.[6] Successful atrial activation mapping depends on several factors, such as the inducibility of tachycardia at the time of EP testing, a stable tachycardia cycle length, the density of

mapping sites, and the selection of an appropriate electrical reference point.

Before starting activation mapping, a time reference point, or so-called fiducial point, should be determined. The ideal fiducial time maker should be distinctive, stable, or consistent. Usually, the onset of the P wave of the AT in the surface electrocardiogram or the electrogram recorded from the CS ostium or high right atrium is a choice. Local activation times are generally measured from the onset of the first rapid deflection of the bipolar electrogram recorded by the distal electrode pair of the mapping catheter to the time-reference point. Once an area of early local activation is found, small movements of the catheter tip in the target region are undertaken until the site is identified with the earliest possible local activation. Simultaneous recording with bipolar pairs distal and proximal from an ablation catheter is helpful in that if the proximal pair has a more attractive electrogram than the distal pair, the catheter may be withdrawn slightly to achieve the same position for the distal electrode. In the area of earliest atrial activation, a low-amplitude, fractionated electrogram in the bipolar recording, coincident with a rapid negative deflection of a QS complex in the unipolar recording, is usually present (**Fig. 3**).

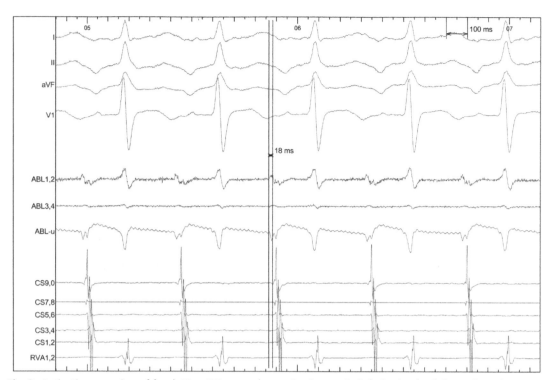

Fig. 3. Activation mapping of focal AT at 450 ms and negative P wave in inferior leads of the surface electrocardiogram. Biatrial activation mapping suggested focal origin and unveiled the earliest atrial activation near the ostium of the CS. The activation at this site (as illustrated by bipolar and unipolar recordings from the ablation catheter [ABL1,2 vs ABL-u]) preceded the proximal CS (CS9–10) by 18 ms. Note that the bipolar signal at the earliest site is fractionated. The sweep speed was 100 mm/s. RVA, right ventricular apex.

In patients who have undergone previous AF ablation, especially those with persistent AF, the mechanisms of macroreentrant ATs are usually (1) mitral isthmus dependent flutter (perimitral AT); (2) roof-dependent flutter; and (3) cavotricuspid isthmus (CTI)–dependent flutter. Using conventional activation mapping based on left atrial and CS activation patterns, these 3 types of AT can be diagnosed quickly.[6] If the left atrial activation pattern is septal to lateral posteriorly and lateral to septal anteriorly (or vice versa), counterclockwise (or clockwise) perimitral AT is the most likely possibility (**Fig. 4**). The activation pattern on the posterior wall is easily determined from the CS recording. If the left atrial activation pattern is septal to lateral both anteriorly and posteriorly and the anterior and posterior walls activate high to low and low to high (or vice versa), respectively, roof-dependent AT rotating counterclockwise (or clockwise) around the antrum of right pulmonary veins is the most likely possibility. If the left atrial activation pattern is lateral to septal both anteriorly and posteriorly and the anterior and posterior walls activate low to high and high to low (or vice versa), respectively, roof-dependent AT rotating counterclockwise (or clockwise) around the antrum of left pulmonary

veins is the most likely possibility. From the therapeutic standpoint, the authors do not need to categorize the roof-dependent circuit as right or left (**Fig. 5**). The left atrial activation pattern in typical counterclockwise CTI-dependent flutter would be septal to lateral and low to high both on the anterior and posterior walls. This possibility would be greatly enhanced if the atrial electrogram recorded from the CTI is earlier than the electrogram recorded from the CS ostium during AT and evidence indicates this type of AT in the 12-lead electrocardiogram.

ENTRAINMENT MAPPING

Entrainment mapping is one of the most powerful tools in EP laboratories. This mapping method can (1) confirm reentry as the underlying mechanism of a sustained arrhythmia, (2) locate an underlying reentrant circuit, and (3) identify the critical isthmus of the reentrant circuit.[7]

Important Concepts

Entrainment

By definition, entrainment is continuous resetting of a reentrant circuit with an excitable gap by a train

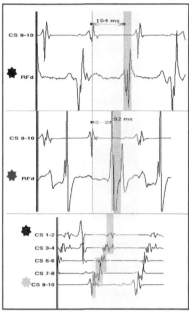

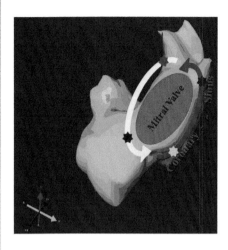

Fig. 4. Atrial activation around the mitral annulus is shown during perimitral AT. A septal (*green marker*) to lateral (*black marker*) atrial activation pattern is seen on the decapolar CS catheter. The mapping catheter positioned at the anterolateral mitral annulus (*red marker*) is activated 92 ms after the proximal CS (reference). The mapping catheter positioned at the anteroseptal mitral annulus (*blue marker*) is activated 154 ms after the proximal CS. Thus, during tachycardia, atrial activation proceeds laterally from the septum in the posterior left atrium and septally from the lateral aspect of the anterior left atrium. This pattern conforms to that of perimitral flutter. The activation pattern around the mitral annulus spans the entire cycle length of this flutter (*orange* pillars march through the *yellow* background that represents one cycle length). The red arrow means from right to left; the green arrow means from anterior to posterior; and the blue arrow means from caudal to cranial. (*Adapted from* Shah AJ, Jadidi A, Liu X, et al. Atrial tachycardias arising from ablation of atrial fibrillation: a proarrhythmic bump or an antiarrhythmic turn? Cardiol Res Pract 2010;2010:950763; with permission.)

of capturing stimuli. During pacing from a site outside the reentry circuit, an appropriately timed stimulus produces a wave of excitation that propagates to the reentry circuit and depolarizes part of the circuit during this excitable gap. The wave then begins propagating in 2 directions in the circuit. The antidromic wave propagates in the reverse direction compared with the reentry circuit wavefronts, and is extinguished when it collides with a previous orthodromic wavefront. The stimulated orthodromic wave follows the path of the previous reentry circuit waves and resets the reentry circuit, continuing the tachycardia.[7,8]

The presence of entrainment for an AT is established (when pacing at a rate slightly faster (10–30 ms) than the AT cycle length) by accelerating all P waves or intracardiac electrograms to the pacing rate, with the presence of constant fusion in the surface electrocardiogram or intracardiac electrogram, and resumption of the AT morphology and rate after cessation of pacing.

Manifest or concealed entrainment

During overdrive pacing, manifest entrainment demonstrates surface electrocardiogram evidence of constant fusion at a constant pacing rate, and progressive fusion with incremental-rate pacing. Entrainment with concealed fusion (also called *concealed entrainment*) is defined as entrainment with orthodromic capture and a surface electrocardiogram complex or intracardiac activation sequence identical to that of the tachycardia.

Postpacing interval

The postpacing interval (PPI) is the period from the last pacing stimulus that entrained the tachycardia to the next nonpaced electrogram recorded at the pacing site. The last paced wave propagates to the circuit, then through the reentry circuit, and back to the pacing site. Thus, the PPI is the sum of the conduction time from the pacing site to the circuit, the revolution time through the circuit, and the conduction time from the circuit back to the pacing site. The PPI is an indication of the proximity of the pacing site to the reentry circuit. During entrainment at sites within the reentrant circuit, the required conduction time is the revolution time through the circuit only; thus, the PPI should be equal or very close (within 20–30 ms) to the tachycardia cycle length. When pacing at

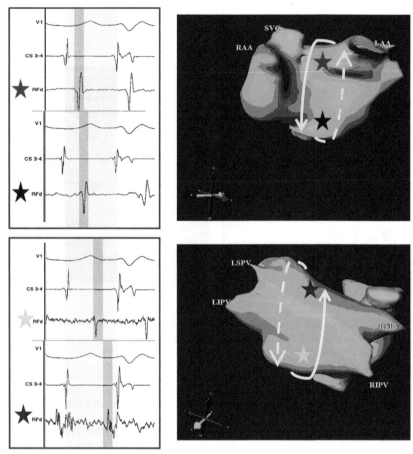

Fig. 5. The electrogram recordings from 4 sites (*red, blue, yellow,* and *maroon stars*) on the anterior and posterior left atrium are timed with a coronary sinus dipole (CS 3–4) as a reference. Local electrograms recorded from the high (*red star*) and low (*blue star*) anterior sites are respectively 168 and 214 ms from the reference suggestive of a high-to-low anterior left atrial activation pattern. Local electrograms recorded from high (*maroon star*) and low (*yellow star*) posterior sites are respectively 274 and 262 ms away from the reference suggestive of a low-to-high posterior left atrial activation pattern. This pattern is consistent with roof-dependent flutter. The red arrow means from right to left; the green arrow means from anterior to posterior; and the blue arrow means from caudal to cranial. (*Adapted from* Shah AJ, Jadidi A, Liu X, et al. Atrial tachycardias arising from ablation of atrial fibrillation: a proarrhythmic bump or an antiarrhythmic turn? Cardiol Res Pract 2010;2010:950763; with permission.)

sites remote from the circuit, the stimulated wavefronts propagate to the circuit, then through the circuit, and finally back to the pacing site. Therefore, the PPI should equal the tachycardia cycle length plus the time required for the stimulus to propagate from the pacing site to the tachycardia circuit and back. The greater the difference between the PPI and the native tachycardia cycle length, the longer the distance between the pacing site and the reentry circuit.

Role of Entrainment Mapping in Interpreting the Mechanism of AT After AF Ablation

In contrast to de novo AT, the prevalence of reentrant ATs is higher in patients with ATs after

AF ablation. Thus, entrainment mapping plays a more important role in the mapping of AT after AF ablation when compared with de novo AT. However, one should keep in mind that the ATs encountered in the context of AF ablation are easy to transform or interrupt during overdrive pacing because of the poor stability of these ATs (resulting from the complexity of the atrial substrate). Therefore, the authors recommend that entrainment maneuvers be guided by the initial activation mapping and be performed at as few sites as possible. For example, confirming the diagnosis with entrainment pacing from 2 opposite segments, such as from septal and lateral sites for perimitral tachycardia or from anterior and posterior walls for roof-dependent macroreentry. In

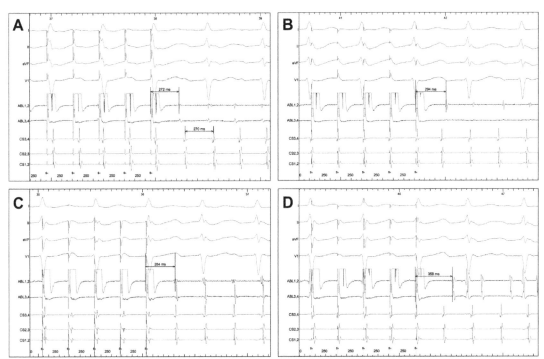

Fig. 6. Entrainment mapping of a roof-dependent atrial tachycardia with cycle length of 270 ms. From top to bottom are the tracings of the surface electrocardiogram (lead I, II, aVF, and V1), and recordings from the distal and proximal electrodes of mapping/ablation catheter (Abl1–2 and Abl3–4) and CS. The electrode pair of CS3–4 was at the ostium of CS, whereas CS1–2 was at the distal CS. During entrainment pacing at a cycle length of 250 ms from the anterior wall (A), the posterior wall (B), and the inferior wall (C) of the left atrium, the PPI minus tachycardia cycle length (TCL) difference are within 30 ms in these 3 sites, indicating that all of the them are in the reentrant circuit, thus supporting the diagnosis of a roof-dependent atrial tachycardia. Considering that the PPI exceeds the TCL by 88 ms when entrainment pacing from the lateral of mitral annuals (D), the possibility of a peri-mitral tachycardia was excluded. The sweep speed was 100 mm/s.

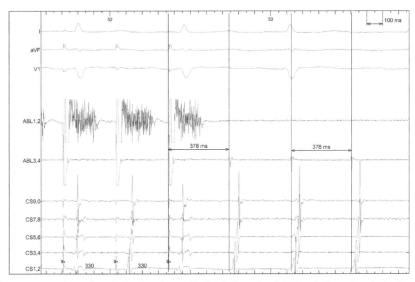

Fig. 7. Entrainment mapping of perimitral tachycardia (cycle length of 376 ms). From top to bottom are tracings of the surface electrogram (lead I, aVF, and V1) and recordings from the distal and proximal electrodes of mapping/ablation catheter (Abl1–2 and Abl3–4) and CS. The electrode pair of CS9–0 was at the ostium of CS, whereas CS1–2 was at the distal CS. During entrainment pacing at a cycle length of 330 ms from the anterior lateral aspect of the mitral annulus, the local electrograms from the pacing site (Abl1–2) were not discernible because of stimulus artifacts; however, the potentials of the proximal electrode pair (Abl3–4) were clear enough to determine the PPI as 378 ms. The sweep speed was 100 mm/s.

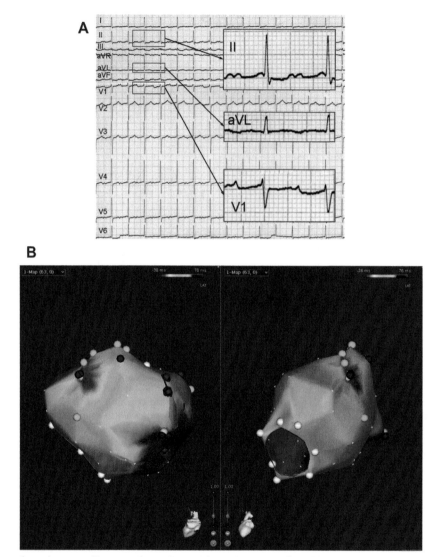

Fig. 8. The surface electrocardiogram of a patient with persistent AT after ablation for paroxysmal AF. (A) During AT, the negative P wave in lead aVL and positive P wave in lead V1 suggest the leftward origin of this tachycardia. The widened and notched P wave in lead V1 and positive P wave in the inferior leads indicate the possible origin of AT at the high lateral aspect of the left atrium. Considering this patient underwent circumferential pulmonary vein isolation only during the index procedure, the most likely origin of this AT was the anterior aspect of the left superior pulmonary vein, which was confirmed by three-dimensional electroanatomic mapping (the site in *red*) and successful ablation at the earliest activation site (B).

addition, long duration of overdrive pacing, especially with high stimulus output, should be avoided to minimize the possibility of AT conversion or interruption. If the difference between the PPI and tachycardia cycle length is less than 30 ms, the pacing site is very close to or lying on the circuit of the reentrant AT. However, if conduction slows in the reentry circuit during pacing, the difference between the PPI and AT cycle length may increase. This phenomenon may occur in patients who are receiving antiarrhythmic medications or after aggressive ablation. In these cases, the PPI may falsely suggest that the pacing site is remote from the circuit. The PPI should be measured for the near-field atrial potential that indicates depolarization of tissue at the pacing site. However, when the electrograms for the pacing site are not discernible because of stimulus artifacts, the timing of the near-field potential for the proximal electrode pair can be related to a consistent intracardiac electrogram or surface electrocardiogram wave to determine the PPI (**Fig. 6**).

Three Deductive Steps

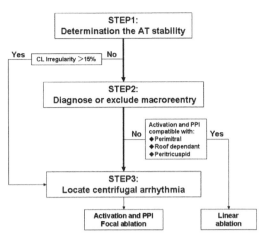

Fig. 9. Stepwise diagnostic algorithm for AT after AT ablation. CL, cycle length.

DIAGNOSTIC MANEUVERS FOR AT AFTER AF ABLATION
Value of a 12-Lead Electrocardiogram

Usually, the P wave morphology in a 12-lead ECG can provide important information in predicting the origin of focal AT after pulmonary vein ablation only (**Fig. 7**).[9] However, the diagnostic and localizing value of the surface electrocardiogram is debatable for ATs arising after aggressive atrial ablation. In this situation, surface P waves no longer provide consistent information on the location of focal AT or mechanisms of reentrant AT, because the magnitude and direction of the vector of atrial activation are tremendously affected by the differential conduction velocity and low-voltage areas of extensively ablated atria.

A Diagnostic Algorithm of AT After AF Ablation Based on Conventional Mapping

Using a conventional mapping strategy based on an understanding of likely mechanisms and locations of ATs, and combining both activation and entrainment mapping, most ATs can be mapped and ablated successfully using a roving ablation catheter and a mapping catheter within the coronary sinus. During ongoing tachycardia, the authors recommend a 3-stepped approach (**Fig. 8**) to diagnose the type of AT after AF ablation.[6]

Step 1: Determine the stability of AT.

Using the electrograms recorded for the left atrial appendage or CS for 1 minute, the mean

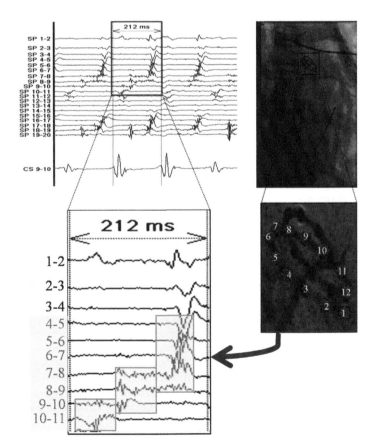

Fig. 10. Example of activation mapping in a patient with localized reentrant AT. Cardiac fluoroscopy in posteroanterior view shows a multipolar spiral catheter (20 mm diameter) and a decapolar catheter. The spiral catheter is mapping left atrial roof. Within a small area of approximately 3 cm², electrical activity spanning across almost the entire cycle length (212 ms) of tachycardia is demonstrated on bipolar electrograms recorded from dipoles 4–5 to 10–11 on the spiral catheter (*yellow* background in the zoom). The electrograms are low voltage with a maximum amplitude of 0.2 mV. This is characteristic of localized reentrant form of focal AT. Instead of a point source, a small area harbors a tiny circuit, which sustains the entire cycle length of a reentrant tachycardia. The remainder of the atria is activated centrifugally, which is consistent with focal tachycardia. (*Adapted from* Shah AJ, Jadidi A, Liu X, et al. Atrial tachycardias arising from ablation of atrial fibrillation: a proarrhythmic bump or an antiarrhythmic turn? Cardiol Res Pract 2010;2010:950763; with permission.)

cycle length and the range of variation in cycle length over 1 minute are assessed. If the variation exceeds 15% of the mean cycle length, a focal mechanism is the most likely diagnosis. However, variation of less than 15% does not rule out the focal mechanism. In the latter situation, the next step is performed to diagnose or rule out macro-reentrant AT.

Step 2: Determine the left atrial activation pattern and entrainment of AT for macroreentry as described in step 1.

Step 3: Localize focal AT or localized reentry.

The atrial activation pattern reflects the direction of centrifugal propagation of AT from the focal source. In a single tachycardia cycle, the activation pattern of CS (proximal to distal or distal to proximal) and the left atrial activation pattern (based on the local activation time of the anterior, posterior, septal, and lateral left atrium) that do not conform to macroreentrant mechanism provide a useful guide for mapping the focal source. A fragmented electrogram spanning 50% to 75% of the tachycardia cycle length may suggest a site of localized small circuit (**Fig. 9**).

The entrainment response for focal AT is characteristically distinct from that of macroreentry. Note that, in contrast to the macroreentrant circuit spread over more than one atrial segment, a small circuit can be localized to one atrial segment only. On entrainment, the PPI continues to decrease as the pacing site approaches the focus. This phenomenon provides an important guide to segmental localization of focal AT.[10–13] A PPI less than 30 ms suggests that the pacing site is near/at the site of interest. It is sometimes difficult to capture at the site of interest even with a high pacing output. In this situation, pacing from an area near the site of interest would yield a PPI within 30 to 50 ms, which is acceptable. Entrainment farther from the proxy site yields a PPI exceeding 50 ms. If the segment of interest cannot be localized to the left atrium according to the AT activation pattern and entrainment criterion, right atrial mapping is performed in the same manner (**Fig. 10**).

SUMMARY

Conventional mapping of AT after AF ablation requires a systematic strategy. Clues regarding the underlying mechanisms of AT can be derived from the P wave morphology of the surface electrocardiogram, the AT cycle length variability, the morphology of unipolar signals, and, more importantly, the atrial activation and entrainment mapping results. Using this systematic mapping strategy, most ATs after AF ablation can be mapped accurately.

REFERENCES

1. Shah AJ, Jadidi A, Liu X, et al. Atrial tachycardias arising from ablation of atrial fibrillation: a proarrhythmic bump or an antiarrhythmic turn? Cardiol Res Pract 2010;2010:950763.
2. Stevenson WG, Soejima K. Recording techniques for clinical electrophysiology. J Cardiovasc Electrophysiol 2005;16:1017–22.
3. Delacretaz E, Soejima K, Gottipaty VK, et al. Single catheter determination of local electrogram prematurity using simultaneous unipolar and bipolar recordings to replace the surface ECG as a timing reference. Pacing Clin Electrophysiol 2001;24:441–9.
4. Stevenson WG. Mapping for localization of target sites. In: Wilber DJ, Packer DL, Stevenson WG, editors. Catheter ablation of cardiac arrhythmias: basic concepts and clinical applications. 3rd edition. Malden (MA): Blackwell Publishing; 2008. p. 49–59.
5. Arora R, Kadish A. Fundamental of intracardiac mapping. In: Huang SK, Wilber DH, editors. Catheter ablation of cardiac arrhythmias. 2nd edition. Philadelphia: WB Saunders; 2011. p. 103–26.
6. Jaïs P, Matsuo S, Knecht S, et al. A deductive mapping strategy for atrial tachycardia following atrial fibrillation ablation: importance of localized reentry. J Cardiovasc Electrophysiol 2009;20:480–91.
7. Waldo AL. Atrial flutter: entrainment characteristics. J Cardiovasc Electrophysiol 1997;8:337–52.
8. Derejko P, Szumowski LJ, Sanders P, et al. Clinical validation and comparison of alternative methods for evaluation of entrainment mapping. J Cardiovasc Electrophysiol 2009;20:741–8.
9. Rajawat YS, Gerstenfeld EP, Patel VV, et al. ECG criteria for localizing the pulmonary vein origin of spontaneous atrial premature complexes: validation using intracardiac recordings. Pacing Clin Electrophysiol 2004;27:182–8.
10. Deo R, Berger R. The clinical utility of entrainment pacing. J Cardiovasc Electrophysiol 2009;20:466–70.
11. Mohamed U, Skanes AC, Gula LJ, et al. A novel pacing maneuver to localize focal atrial tachycardia. J Cardiovasc Electrophysiol 2007;18:1–6.
12. Patel AM, d'Avila A, Neuzil P, et al. Atrial tachycardia after ablation of persistent atrial fibrillation: identification of the critical isthmus with a combination of multielectrode activation mapping and targeted entrainment mapping. Circ Arrhythm Electrophysiol 2008;1:14–22.
13. Weerasooriya R, Jaïs P, Wright M, et al. Catheter ablation of atrial tachycardia following atrial fibrillation ablation. J Cardiovasc Electrophysiol 2009;20:833–8.

Three-Dimensional Invasive Mapping: Focus on Atrial Tachycardias

Shinsuke Miyazaki, MD*, Amir S. Jadidi, MD

KEYWORDS

- Atrial tachycardia • 3D mapping system • Atrial fibrillation • Catheter ablation

KEY POINTS

- The 3-dimensional anatomic mapping system depicts the atrial activation pattern in atrial tachycardia.
- It is essential to have a stable reference, acquire a certain minimum number of points all around the chamber, and accurately annotate double/fragmented/multispike potential.
- Entrainment mapping must be used for confirmation of diagnosis evident from activation maps.
- Simultaneous high-density mapping with a multielectrode catheter facilitates identification of the critical slow conduction zone.

INTRODUCTION

Technologic advances in electroanatomic mapping systems have greatly contributed to the improvement of catheter ablation for complex arrhythmias. Currently, several advanced mapping systems are available, and each system has both advantages and disadvantages. Although it is possible to map atrial tachycardia (AT) post atrial fibrillation (AF) ablation, as described in other articles elsewhere in this issue, a 3-dimensional (3D) anatomic mapping system enables us to visualize the tachycardia circuit directly. In this article, we describe the additional utility of a 3D mapping system for AT post AF ablation.

CARTO MAPPING SYSTEM

The Carto mapping system (Biosense Webster, Diamond Bar, CA) is one of the most extensively used 3D mapping systems. The system uses ultra–low-intensity magnetic fields emitted from a locator pad beneath the laboratory table. The magnetic field strength is detected by a location sensor embedded proximal to the tip of a specialized mapping catheter. The geometry is used to display electrical information, such as activation sequence or local electrogram amplitude, which is simultaneously recorded at each catheter position. The anatomic accuracy of the system is less than 1 mm. It can also show the tip of the ablation catheter moving within the 3D image. Use of this image to guide mapping and ablation minimizes fluoroscopic exposure. Tagging the sites with interesting electrogram information helps to proceed further and analyze the mechanism of the tachycardia.

Activation Mapping

The activation map is constructed using a stable timing reference electrogram. Selection of a stable and reliable timing reference is critical for efficient and successful mapping. The reference electrogram, typically a coronary sinus bipole, should be chosen such that there are no confusing far-field components.

Conflicts of Interest: None.
Disclosures: None.
Arrhythmology Department, Hôpital Cardiologique du Haut-Lévêque, Université Victor Segalen Bordeaux II, Avenue de Magellan, Bordeaux, Pessac Cedex 33604, France
* Corresponding author. Hôpital Haut Lévêque, Avenue de Magellan, Bordeaux, Pessac 33604, France.
E-mail address: mshinsuke@k3.dion.ne.jp

Card Electrophysiol Clin 5 (2013) 153–160
http://dx.doi.org/10.1016/j.ccep.2013.01.007
1877-9182/13/$ – see front matter © 2013 Elsevier Inc. All rights reserved.

Before creating a detailed 3D map of an arrhythmia, the electrophysiologist should have a reasonable idea as to where (in which cardiac chamber) the tachycardia source or circuit is located. Most of the ATs post AF ablation arise in the left atrium; some are from the right atrium. Entrainment pacing is useful for accurately locating the chamber. Assuming that the reference bipole is stable and the window of interest and tachycardia cycle length remain unchanged, the consistency in the annotation of electrograms recorded on the roving mapping catheter determines the diagnostic accuracy of the mapping process. It is important to acquire a certain minimum number of points all around the chamber to have reliable diagnosis from the maps created. Otherwise, there could be large gaps between the collected data points.

The operator must have a consistent plan as to how to time the electrogram with its reference, as well as a method of handling double potentials and fragmented signals because the annotation of these potentials is the key to create an accurate activation map. Two distinct electrograms separated by an isoelectric interval (double potentials) can be recorded from a catheter on either a line of conduction block or conduction delay and represent electrical activation on both sides of such a line. It is generally unacceptable to simply take the earliest signal when double potentials are present because depending on the selection of mapping window and catheter position, it may or may not always be the near-field (local) signal. One of the double potentials has to be the far-field electrogram. Identifying the near-field electrogram and differentiating it from the far-field electrograms are crucial steps. Thus, on one side of the line of block/delay, the near-field signal may be the second component of double potential, whereas the same signal becomes far-field when recorded from the opposite side of the line of block. If such identification is challenging, it is better to tag such a site as "double potential for location only."

Fragmented signals are multicomponent signals without isoelectric intervals between components. These are often areas of slow conduction, and individual components may reflect local or far-field activation. These sites may represent a slow zone of conduction for the given tachycardia or bystander areas of slow conduction that may require iterative ablation for complete substrate modification. Sites of fragmented signals may be initially tagged as location-only points without assigned activation time because it is not usually possible to determine the near-field component indicating local activation, especially when the signal is low-amplitude with long duration. It should be remembered, however, for reentry tachycardias, the complete cycle length of the tachycardia will not be seen in an otherwise appropriate map in the correct chamber of origin when the fractionated "location-only" points are in the reentry circuit. After complete mapping of the chamber, the electrophysiologist should look back at tagged fragmented signal sites to determine which of these is likely to represent the slow zone for the given circuit. This can usually be determined by reviewing the wave front of activation at adjacent regions. Inclusion of the appropriate region in the map, then, may account for the remaining portion of the tachycardia cycle length.

Macroreentrant AT and Focal AT

A hallmark of macroreentrant AT is the presence of areas of early activation adjacent to late regions. That is, the earliest site meets the latest site (**Figs. 1–3**). It is necessary to account for at least 90% of the tachycardia cycle length to visualize a reentrant circuit. Typically if less than 50% of the tachycardia cycle length is accounted for by mapping one atrium, the circuit is probably contained in the contralateral atrium (**Fig. 4**). On the contrary, focal arrhythmias show the pattern in which the earliest activation site is surrounded concentrically by those with subsequent activation (**Fig. 5**). The activation map typically spans less than 60% of the tachycardia cycle length, and the latest site usually does not meet the earliest site.

Substrate Mapping

A 3D mapping system also enables substrate mapping. A substrate map is a compilation of the voltage amplitudes of all contact points with the mapping catheter in a cardiac chamber. A coded color range is assigned that indicates the peak-to-peak amplitude of the signal. By adjusting this color scale manually, the operator can visualize areas of low voltage and compare these sites with scar and relatively normal myocardium. Critical to accurate substrate mapping is obtaining adequate electrode-tissue contact when cataloging the voltages from the derived signals. Combining fluoroscopy, intracardiac echocardiography, and analysis of the near-field components of the signal must be carefully executed to create a valid substrate map. Usually substrate mapping is used for catheter ablation of ventricular tachycardia, and might be helpful for catheter ablation of unmappable multiple ATs.

Pitfalls

An important caveat with electroanatomic mapping is that the catheter tip must be in good contact with the endocardial surface for each

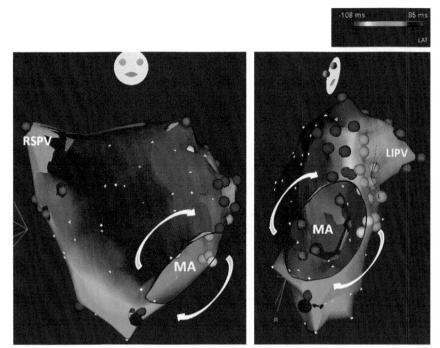

Fig. 1. Left atrial activation map during clockwise peri-mitral AT with a cycle length of 210 ms. Tachycardia cycle length is mostly covered by the activation map. White arrows indicate the activation sequence of the tachycardia. LIPV, left inferior pulmonary vein; MA, mitral annulus; RSPV, right superior pulmonary vein.

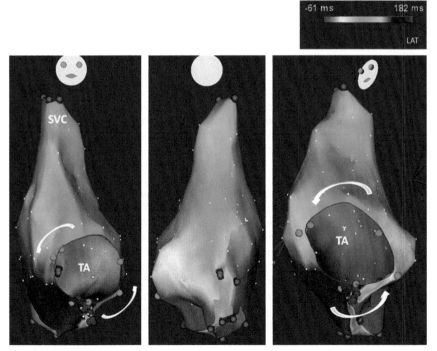

Fig. 2. Right atrial activation map during common (counterclockwise) atrial flutter with a cycle length of 260 ms. Tachycardia cycle length is mostly covered by the activation map. White arrows indicate the activation sequence of the tachycardia. SVC, superior vena cava; TA, tricuspid annulus.

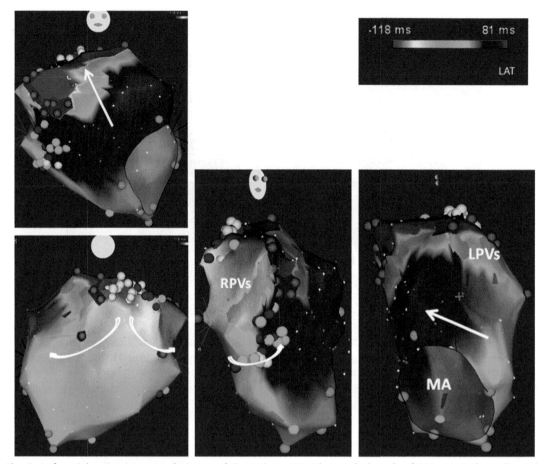

Fig. 3. Left atrial activation map during roof-dependent AT with a cycle length of 210 ms. Tachycardia cycle length is mostly covered by the activation map. White arrows indicate the activation sequence of the tachycardia. LPVs: left pulmonary veins; MA, mitral annulus; RPVs, right pulmonary veins.

electrogram collected. Failure to recognize poor contact could result in collection of phantom data points, suggesting low-amplitude scar, when, in fact, the catheter tip may be simply floating in the atrial cavity. A newly developed contact sensor catheter could resolve this problem.

A limitation of this system is that tachycardia must remain stable for the duration of data acquisition. A newly developed system that acquires multiple points simultaneously would shorten the mapping duration. It is not well suited for mapping unstable ATs because the current system acquires point-by-point information. If the tachycardia shifts repeatedly during the mapping, the sinus rhythm map can be examined to identify the most likely narrow conduction corridors. By displaying an atrial voltage map, areas of scar can be identified to permit the localization of channels that form potential reentrant circuits.

If highly fractionated and/or wide potentials, including multiple components, are present, it might be difficult to assign an activation time. In such a case, reentrant arrhythmia might be confused with focal rhythm. As described previously, careful annotation is required for these potentials. If linear lesions were created previously, the influence of the linear lesion on the activation map should be considered.

In comparison with the simple AT, multiple different ATs are frequently encountered in the context of AF ablation, which would require long procedure time for creating multiple AT maps. Multiple ATs may coexist. The single activation map of these ATs is very complex, and requires careful mapping for reaching a precise diagnosis.

Prior studies[1,2] demonstrated that localized ATs were commonly observed in the context of AF ablation. Because localized ATs cover most of the tachycardia cycle length in a small area, precise annotation is challenging (**Fig. 6**). A small error in annotation could completely change the global activation map.

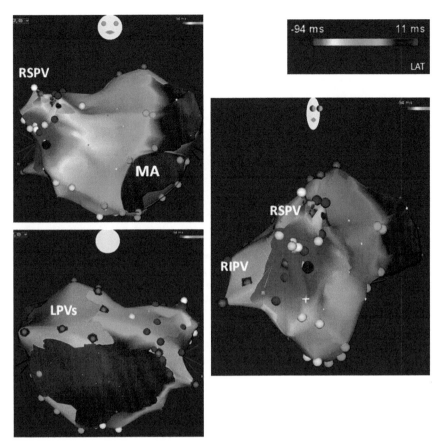

Fig. 4. Left atrial activation map during focal AT with a cycle length of 190 ms arising from mid posterior right atrium. The tachycardia cycle length is not entirely covered and the map suggested focal activation pattern. The earliest activation site is the left septum; therefore, the right atrium should be mapped sequentially. LPV, left pulmonary vein; MA, mitral annulus; RIPV, right inferior pulmonary vein; RSPV, right superior pulmonary vein.

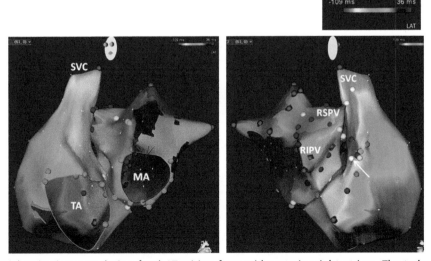

Fig. 5. Bi-atrial activation map during focal AT arising from mid posterior right atrium. The tachycardia cycle length is not entirely covered and the map suggested focal activation pattern. The Carto map clarified the anatomic relationship of 2 chambers. The tachycardia was terminated by the application at the site with white tag (*white arrow*). MA, mitral annulus; RIPV, right inferior pulmonary vein; RSPV, right superior pulmonary vein; SVC, superior vena cava; TA, tricuspid annulus.

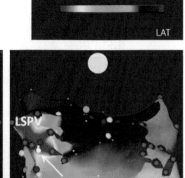

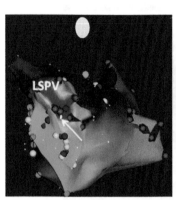

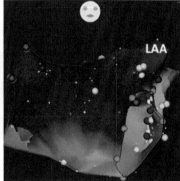

Fig. 6. Left atrial activation map during localized reentrant AT with a cycle length of 340 ms at left mitral isthmus. The tachycardia was terminated by the application at the site with the white tag (*white arrow*). Most of the tachycardia cycle length was covered on the mapping catheter at this site. LAA, left atrial appendage; LSPV, left superior pulmonary vein.

ENSITE NAVX MAPPING SYSTEM
Simultaneous High-Density Multielectrode Mapping

The Ensite NavX Velocity Mapping system (St. Jude Medical, St. Paul, MN) enables creation of high-density electroanatomic maps using multielectrode catheters for map acquisition. Suitable multielectrode catheters that enable high resolution and rapid atrial mapping are circumferential single-loop and double-loop catheters (eg, Optima, SJM [St. Jude Medical, St. Paul, MN]; AFocus HD II double loop, SJM; Lasso, BW [BW, Diamond Bar, CA]), as well as the multispline catheter PentaRay (BW, Diamond Bar, CA). High-density atrial maps can be acquired using either the double-loop circumferential catheters or the PentaRay (BW) catheter within 8 ± 3 minutes.[3,4] Because of the smaller electrode size (1 mm) when compared with an RF ablation catheter (3.5 to 4.0 mm), recorded electrograms have a high local resolution and contain less far-field components. Additionally, with a single acquisition at a given catheter position, up to 20 bipolar electrograms (originating from the whole catheter-tissue contact area) can be added to the electrical map, thus displaying the regional activation of the mapped chamber (**Fig. 7**). To exclude acquisition of far-field (nonlocal) electrograms, the distance of

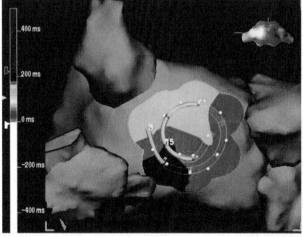

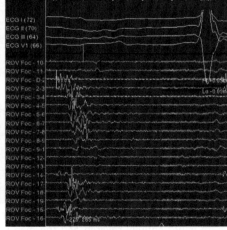

Fig. 7. Simultaneous multielectrode mapping with the NavX Velocity System. A single acquisition using the double-loop circumferential catheter (AFocus HDII, SJMed) enables regional mapping over 5 cm² of the left atrial roof.

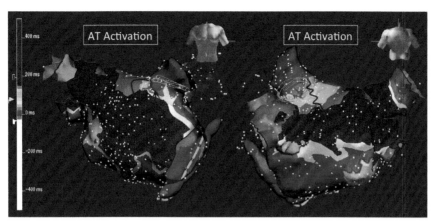

Fig. 8. A localized reentrant tachycardia at the junction of the left atrial roof and left atrial appendage with high density of isochrones (= slow conduction) in that region. The tachycardia was terminated by ablation at the site where blue, purple, white, and red isochrones meet. The black arrow in left panel illustrates the region of localized reentry circuit (1.5 cm diameter), that displays all colours of the AT activation map (*purple, white, redyellow, and blue*) corresponding to the entire AT cycle length. The black arrow in the right panel illustrates the region of slow conduction with isochrone shrinkage at posterior left atrial wall, that is part of the AT critical isthmus.

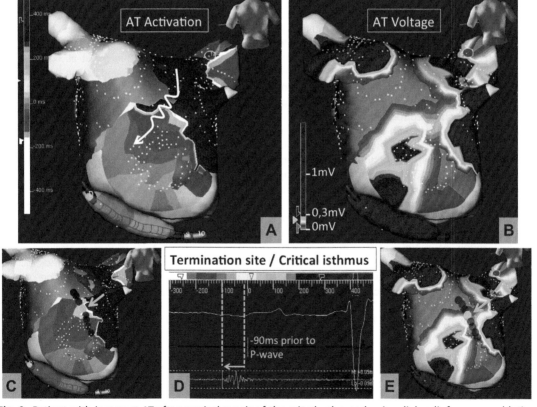

Fig. 9. Patient with incessant AT after surgical repair of the mitral valve and epicardial radiofrequency ablation for chronic atrial fibrillation. High-density activation (*A*) and voltage (*B*) maps of a reentrant circuit using a channel (*white arrow* in [*A*]) between 2 regions of scar at the posterior left atrium. The successful ablation site at the critical slow conduction isthmus (within the channel) shows isochrone shrinkage and a fractionated potential (*D*), that precedes beginning of P-wave by 90 ms. Note that the electrograms in the channel have low voltage (<0.3 mV). See light green marker and arrow in At activation map (*C*) and At voltage map (*E*).

recorded signals from the geometry surface is calculated by the system and the operator can choose the maximum distance at which acquired electrograms are included to the electrical map (for activation map <8 mm and for accurate voltage mapping <3 mm). This distance (electrogram projection distance to geometry surface) can also be modified after acquisition of the total map.

Visualization of Slow Conduction Sites and Critical Isthmuses on NavX Maps

Identification of critical slow conduction sites is crucial to establish the diagnosis and enable successful ablation of reentrant tachycardia circuits. The NavX maps create isochronal maps that enable spatial visualization of the slow conduction isthmuses, responsible for maintenance of reentrant tachycardia. The regions with highest regional isochrone density showing "isochrone shrinkage" are the critical sites of slow conduction. **Fig. 8** demonstrates a localized reentrant tachycardia at the junction of the left atrial roof and left atrial appendage with high density of isochrones in the region of slow conduction. The tachycardia was terminated by ablation at the site where purple, white, and red isochrones meet. During multielectrode mapping, special care has to be paid to how each electrogram is annotated. False annotation of electrograms from both the reference or mapping catheter leads to acquisition of not a single false-annotated electrogram to the map, but up to 20 "bad" electrograms. Therefore, only clear tachycardia beats with correct annotation of the reference and mapping electrograms should be included in the map. False annotations should be corrected immediately during the mapping process to create a high-density map that is useful for diagnosis and treatment of tachycardia.

Fig. 9 demonstrates isochronal (**Fig. 9**A) and voltage (**Fig. 9**B) maps in a patient who underwent surgical repair of mitral valve combined with epicardial RF ablation for chronic atrial fibrillation. The isochronal map in **Fig. 9**A shows the slow conduction "channel" with isochrone shrinkage in the region of low voltage (<0.3 mV). The critical channel is located between the gray areas of complete scar (peak-to-peak bipolar voltage <0.05 mV). The electrogram at the site of AT termination (see **Fig. 9**D) shows presystolic/diastolic activity (–90 ms before beginning of P-wave). Ablation at that site (green lesion markers in **Fig. 9**C, E) terminated atrial tachycardia after 1 minute of RF delivery. However, a linear lesion connecting the 2 scar areas (gray regions) to each other was necessary to cut the more than1-cm-wide channel. After a follow-up period of 15 months, the patient has remained free from recurrence of AT.

SUMMARY

Identification of critical slow conduction sites is crucial for the diagnosis and successful ablation of reentrant tachycardia circuits. This may be especially difficult in patients having extensive scar regions with wide areas of low and fractionated electrograms (see **Fig. 9**). High-resolution multielectrode mapping enables creation of electroanatomic maps with identification of scar regions and spatial width of underlying critical isthmuses in patients with reentrant scar-related tachycardia.

REFERENCES

1. Shah D, Sunthorn H, Burri H, et al. Narrow, slow-conducting isthmus dependent left atrial reentry developing after ablation for atrial fibrillation: ECG characterization and elimination by focal RF ablation. J Cardiovasc Electrophysiol 2006;17(5):508–15.
2. Jaïs P, Matsuo S, Knecht S, et al. A deductive mapping strategy for atrial tachycardia following atrial fibrillation ablation: importance of localized reentry. J Cardiovasc Electrophysiol 2009;20(5):480–91.
3. Jadidi AS, Duncan E, Miyazaki S, et al. Functional nature of electrogram fractionation demonstrated by left atrial high-density mapping. Circ Arrhythm Electrophysiol 2012;5(1):32–42.
4. Patel AM, d'Avila A, Neuzil P, et al. Atrial tachycardia after ablation of persistent atrial fibrillation: identification of the critical isthmus with a combination of multielectrode activation mapping and targeted entrainment mapping. Circ Arrhythm Electrophysiol 2008; 1(1):14–22.

Practical Mapping Algorithm
An Overview of the Bordeaux Approach

Yuki Komatsu, MD*, Pierre Jais, MD

KEYWORDS

- Atrial tachycardia • Mapping • Activation • Macroreentry • Focal AT

KEY POINTS

- The ablation of atrial tachycardia (AT) in the context of persistent atrial fibrillation ablation is often the final indispensable step toward long-term maintenance of sinus rhythm.
- Deductive mapping approach of ATs is based on up to 3 steps: (1) determination of cycle length regularity, (2) diagnosis or exclusion of macroreentry, and (3) localization of focal AT.
- If cycle length variability is greater than 15%, a focal AT is deemed likely.
- A reference channel is placed close to the mapping catheter channel to clearly delineate the AT cycle length window, allowing the operator to know immediately which parts (early, mid, or late) of the cycle have been mapped.
- To minimize the risk of interruption of AT, entrainment maneuvers as guided by the activation mapping have to be performed as few times as possible.

INTRODUCTION

Catheter ablation is becoming a successful treatment option for persistent atrial fibrillation (AF) with electrogram-based ablation and linear ablation after pulmonary vein (PV) isolation.[1–8] Such extensive ablation is highly associated with the occurrence of atrial tachycardia (AT) during the index procedure or later during follow-up.[2] The incidence of AT is 40% to 57% in patients undergoing PV isolation combined with electrogram-based atrial ablation and linear ablation.[9–12] It is often difficult to prevent and manage these ATs by antiarrhythmic medications. In addition, they are more symptomatic than persistent AF. The ablation of AT in the context of persistent AF ablation is often the final indispensable step toward long-term maintenance of sinus rhythm.[2] Elimination of ATs is associated with the long-term maintenance of sinus rhythm.[13] However, mapping and ablation of these ATs are challenging, because

they have unpredictable and often complex mechanisms and they can frequently be multiple. In this article, an overview of the practical approaches to the treatment of AT in the context of persistent AF ablation is presented.

DEFINITIONS OF AT

AT is characterized by a monomorphic P wave with a consistent intracardiac activation sequence, and is classified into the following 3 categories; in the context of persistent AF ablation, these definitions of AT mechanisms are used (**Fig. 1**).

1. Macro reentry is defined as a circuit involving more than 3 atrial segments, usually greater than 2 cm in diameter and in which more than 75% of the circuit is mapped.
2. Focal source tachycardia is defined as centrifugal activation originating from a discrete site that gathers automaticity, triggered activity,

Conflicts of Interest: None.
Disclosures: None.
Hôpital Cardiologique du Haut-Lévêque, Université Victor Segalen Bordeaux II, Avenue de Magellan, Bordeaux, Pessac 33604, France
* Corresponding author.
E-mail address: yk.komat@gmail.com

cardiacEP.theclinics.com

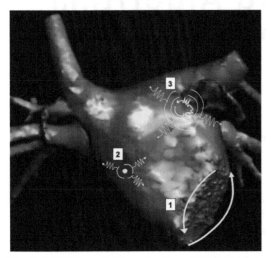

Fig. 1. Definition of AT mechanisms. (1) Macroreentrant tachycardia, (2) Focal source tachycardia, (3) Localized reentrant tachycardia. Yellow arrows indicate the activation directions.

and reentrant mechanisms, in which less than 75% of the cycle can be mapped in the region of interest.

3. Localized reentry constitutes a circuit involving 1 or 2 adjacent segments, usually smaller than 2 cm in diameter and spanning more than 75% of the cycle length within the involved segments.

Approximately 46% of ATs after stepwise ablation of persistent AF are macroreentrant.[14] Among

those ATs, the most frequent are perimitral circuits (58%), followed by roof-dependent circuits (30%) and peritricuspid circuits (5%). Among focal ATs (54% of total ATs), localized reentry is the most frequent mechanism, representing 71% of focal ATs (37% of total ATs). As a rule of thumb, macro-reentrant AT is easy to diagnose but more difficult to treat, whereas focal and localized reentrant ATs are difficult to map but easier to eliminate.

DEDUCTIVE MAPPING STEPS

At the outset, it is important to know about previously ablated sites and whether bidirectional block was achieved or not, if linear ablation was performed. For mapping and diagnosis of AT, we adopt the following 3-stepped approach (**Fig. 2**).[14]

Step 1: Determination of Stability of AT Cycle Length

Assessment of AT cycle length stability is the first step in deductive mapping strategy. The regularity (stability) of a given AT is assessed using dedicated in-built software. Up to 30 tachycardia cycles recorded on the decapolar catheter in the coronary sinus (CS) or the mapping catheter in the left appendage are usually selected. When AT cycle length varies by more than 15%, a focal source mechanism with centrifugal atrial activation is deemed highly likely (**Fig. 3**A). In this situation, the macroreentrant mechanism is unlikely. However, when AT

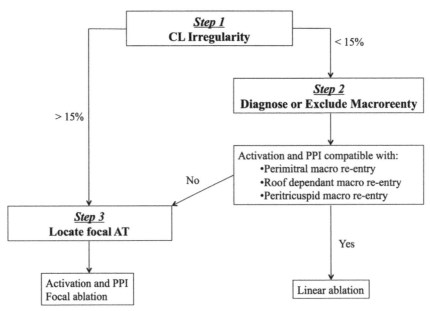

Fig. 2. Deductive mapping steps. Three deductive steps for mapping and ablation of AT in the context of persistent AF ablation.

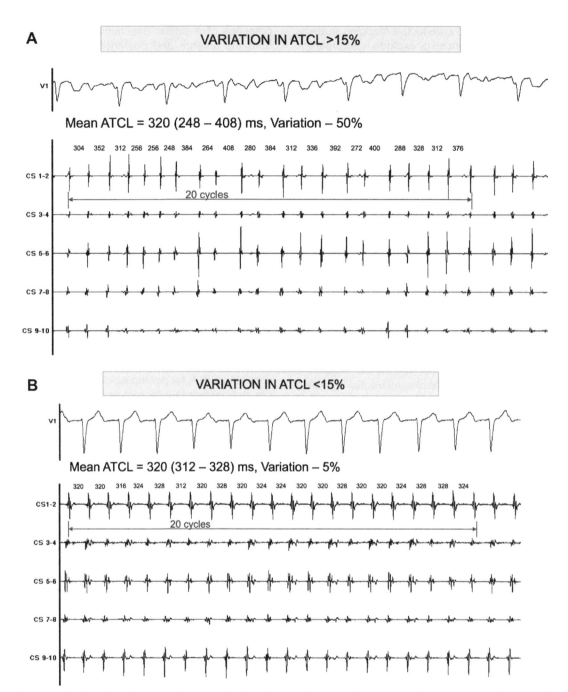

Fig. 3. Cycle length variation. When AT cycle length varies by more than 15%, a focal source mechanism with centrifugal atrial activation is deemed highly likely, and the macroreentrant mechanism is not considered as a possibility (*A*). When the AT cycle length variation is less than 15%, both macroreentry and focal source with centrifugal atrial activation are the possible mechanisms of tachycardia (*B*).

cycle length variation is less than 15%, both macroreentry and focal source with centrifugal atrial activation are the possible mechanisms of tachycardia (see **Fig. 3**B).

Step 2: Diagnosis or Exclusion of Macroreentry

If AT cycle length variation is less than 15%, activation and entrainment mapping are undertaken as the second step in deductive mapping strategy. The aim is to diagnose or exclude macroreentry. In principle, macroreentrant tachycardia causes activation of some part of the atrium during a given instant in the AT cycle length window. A fixed AT cycle length window is provided by the discrete atrial signal recorded by CS catheter and used as a reference. Macroreentrant AT represents 1 of the following 3 (**Fig. 4**): (1) Mitral isthmus–dependent flutter (perimitral AT), (2) Roof-dependent flutter, and (3) Cavotricuspid isthmus–dependent flutter (peritricuspid AT). The atrial sites around the mitral annulus (MA), the pulmonary venous antra, and the tricuspid annulus are mapped to look for the presence of activity during 1 tachycardia cycle length.

1. Perimitral Flutter

In perimitral reentry, opposite locations on the MA cannot be activated simultaneously. The activation wavefront spanning all of the cycle length can be followed along the MA (**Fig. 5**). Recognition of this wavefront is critical for the diagnosis of perimitral reentry. Perimitral reentry is suspected based on the sequential circumferential activation of lateral and septal regions around the anterior MA in addition to the CS activations (which represent posterior MA activation). In the presence of either distal to proximal activation recorded by the CS catheter or vice versa, perimitral reentrant AT is possible (see **Fig. 5**). If the sequential activation does not go around the MA, perimitral reentry can be excluded.

2. Roof-dependent reentry

If perimitral reentry is ruled out, roof-dependent macroreentry is mapped for along the longitudinal axis of the left atrium (LA). In roof-dependent macroreentry, the LA is activated from the roof toward the annulus or otherwise in the anterior wall and in the reverse direction on the posterior wall (**Fig. 6**). No 2 locations on the opposite segments can be activated simultaneously, and

presence of a similar direction of activation on both the anterior and posterior walls rules out roof-dependent flutter.

3. Peritricuspid Reentry

In peritricuspid reentry, the CS is activated from proximal to distal, and both the anterior and posterior MA can be activated almost simultaneously. The activation mapping along the tricuspid annulus covers all of the AT cycle length.

Entrainment maneuvers

Entrainment maneuvers to confirm the diagnosis of macroreentrant AT should be performed in 2 opposite segments to minimize the risk of disorganization or interruption of tachycardia. The selection of pacing sites is guided by the activation map (ie, septum and mitral isthmus regions for perimitral or anterior and posterior wall for roof-dependent macroreentry). After the AT is entrained from 2 opposite atrial segments for the suspected type of macroreentry (eg, septal and lateral LA for perimitral flutter; septal and lateral right atrium [RA] for peritricuspid flutter; and anterior and posterior LA for roof-dependent flutter), if the postpacing interval (PPI) is greater than 30 milliseconds in any 1 of the pairs of opposite segments, macroreentry is ruled out and focal tachycardia remains the only possible diagnosis, leading to step 3.

Step 3: Location of Focal Arrhythmia

After adequately ruling out the possibility of macroreentry in a stable AT, localization of focal source is undertaken as the last step of deductive mapping strategy. If the variation in AT cycle length is more than 15%, localization of focal source is undertaken without considering the possibility of macroreentry. Activation mapping is performed in the LA followed by, if required, the RA to look for the site of earliest activation with a fixed reference electrogram. The preferential

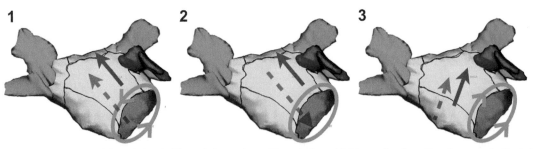

Fig. 4. Macroreentry: (1) perimitral; (2) roof-dependent; (3) peritricuspid. The activation directions are indicated by the red and orange arrows.

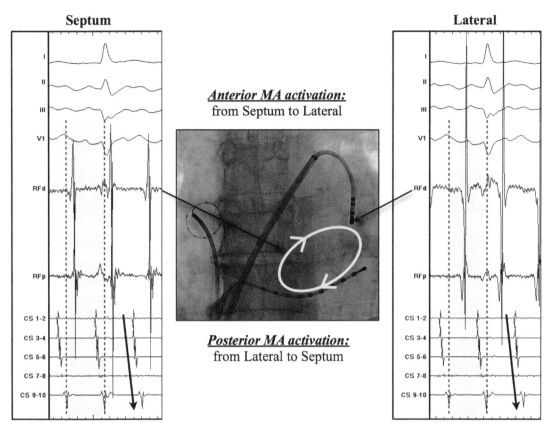

Fig. 5. Perimitral reentry. The signals of the CS show distal to proximal activation sequence, which implies that the activation occurs from lateral to septum on the posterior MA. The CS timing reference is marked by the red dotted lines. The activation of the anterior septum is earlier than that of the anterior lateral, which implies that the activation occurs from septum to lateral on the anterior MA. The activation pattern around the MA, as indicated by the direction of yellow arrows, is consistent with perimitral reentry. The entrainment maneuvers at 2 opposite sites (the septum and lateral) confirmed the diagnosis (not shown).

regions for focal AT are shown in **Fig. 7**. The PV-LA junction, base of LA appendage, and LA septum are the regions with high incidences of focal origin ATs.

The activation pattern of the CS provides a useful guide for initial mapping to the septal side (proximal to distal CS activation) or the lateral side of the LA (distal to proximal CS activation). The conventional ablation catheter is then used to search for a region showing centrifugal activation. By using a fixed timing reference to permit exploration of the AT cycle length window, the activation sequence is recorded (**Fig. 8**). In addition, areas showing a fragmented electrogram spanning more than 50% of tachycardia cycle length are regions suggestive of localized reentry. They are noted for subsequent analysis using an entrainment maneuver. PPI of less than 30 milliseconds suggests that the pacing site is near the site of interest.[14,15]

Ablation

Focal ATs are ablated at the site of origin. Radiofrequency energy with power of up to 30 W and a target temperature up to 42°C is delivered via an irrigated tip catheter. If tachycardia fails to terminate or convert to another tachycardia after at least 60 seconds of energy delivery, the site is deemed unsatisfactory and further mapping is performed to localize a better site for ablation. Macroreentrant AT is targeted by performing linear ablation. Linear ablation of the LA roof is performed by joining the ostia of 2 isolated superior PVs at the most cranial aspect of the LA. Perimitral flutter is targeted by performing linear ablation at the mitral isthmus. Ablation of the mitral isthmus is performed by withdrawing the catheter from the ventricular side of the mitral isthmus (where the atrial/ventricular electrogram ratio is 1:1 or 2:1) to the isolated left inferior PV. Ablation within the CS on the epicardial side of the mitral isthmus

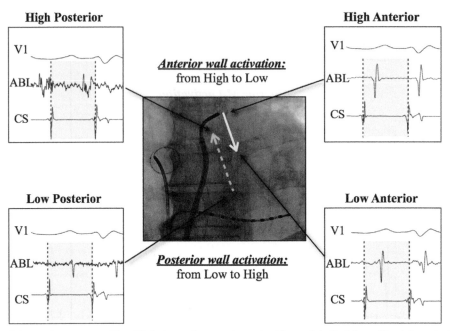

High Posterior

Anterior wall activation:
from High to Low

High Anterior

Low Posterior

Posterior wall activation:
from Low to High

Low Anterior

Fig. 6. Roof-dependent reentry. The CS timing reference is marked by red dotted lines. The LA posterior wall is activated from low to high region. The reverse direction of activation (from high to low region) on the anterior wall is consistent with the roof-dependent reentry, as indicated by the direction of yellow arrows. The entrainment maneuvers at 2 sites (the anterior and posterior wall) confirm the diagnosis (not shown).

is performed when bidirectional conduction block cannot be achieved across the isthmus endocardially; this is often necessary. Power of up to 35 W endocardially and up to 20 W epicardially (distally within the CS) is required to achieve transmural lesion. CTI ablation is performed conventionally for CTI-dependent flutters. The end point is creation of complete bidirectional conduction block across the linear lesion. Confirmation of bidirectional block is undertaken after restoration of sinus rhythm.

Confirmation of bidirectional conduction block of linear lesion
Block across the mitral isthmus linear ablation is shown by differential pacing from distal and proximal CS dipoles sequentially and recording the time of activation in the LA appendage. If LA appendage activation is earlier, with proximal CS pacing rather than more distal CS pacing, it is suggestive of unidirectional block. If subsequent pacing from the LA appendage shows that activation in CS proceeds from the proximal dipole

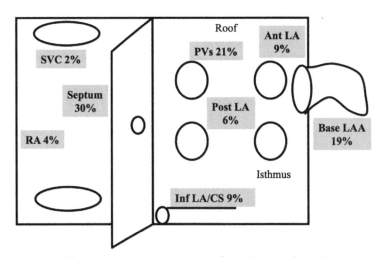

Fig. 7. Preferential regions of focal AT. Ant, anterior; LAA, left atrial appendage; SVC, superior vena cava.

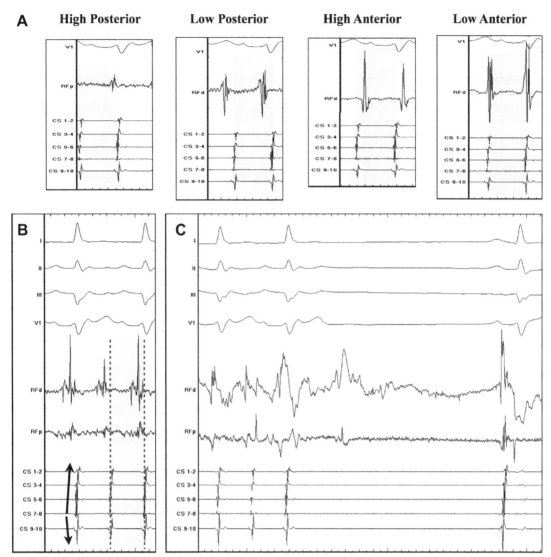

Fig. 8. Focal AT. (*A*) The activation pattern of the CS is unlikely to be perimitral reentry. Similar direction of activation on both walls (from low to high) rules out roof-dependent flutter. (*B*) Among the CS electrodes, CS 7 to 8 is the earliest activation timing. By using a fixed timing reference to permit exploration of the AT cycle length window (*red area*), the earliest activation site is searched for on the low LA posterior wall and septum. Earliest activation site on the low posterior LA has a fractionated signal. (*C*) Ablation at the site terminates the tachycardia.

distally, this is conclusive of bidirectional block. Estimation of block across the roof linear ablation is undertaken in sinus rhythm or LA appendage pacing. If the activation of posterior LA occurs from below upwards, this confirms unidirectional block along the roof line. Subsequent differential pacing on the posterior LA and recording the time of activation in the LA appendage are performed to confirm bidirectional block. LA appendage activation with inferoposterior LA pacing should occur earlier than superoposterior LA pacing to conclude that the roof linear ablation

is bidirectionally blocked. CTI block is confirmed conventionally.

SUMMARY

Post-AF ablation ATs are often multiple, complex, and leave patients in a more symptomatic state than AF. However, they are considered as the last step in the process of persistent AF ablation, in which they are commonly encountered. Their elimination is associated with the long-term maintenance of sinus rhythm. A deductive mapping approach for the diagnosis of ATs with assessment of atrial activation sequence and confirmation by entrainment maneuvers is efficient and rapid.

REFERENCES

1. Cappato R, Calkins H, Chen SA, et al. Updated worldwide survey on the methods, efficacy, and safety of catheter ablation for human atrial fibrillation. Circ Arrhythm Electrophysiol 2010;3:32–8.
2. Haissaguerre M, Sanders P, Hocini M, et al. Catheter ablation of long-lasting persistent atrial fibrillation: critical structures for termination. J Cardiovasc Electrophysiol 2005;16:1125–37.
3. Nademanee K, McKenzie J, Kosar E, et al. A new approach for catheter ablation of atrial fibrillation: mapping of the electrophysiologic substrate. J Am Coll Cardiol 2004;43:2044–53.
4. Willems S, Klemm H, Rostock T, et al. Substrate modification combined with pulmonary vein isolation improves outcome of catheter ablation in patients with persistent atrial fibrillation: a prospective randomized comparison. Eur Heart J 2006;27:2871–8.
5. Oral H, Chugh A, Good E, et al. Radiofrequency catheter ablation of chronic atrial fibrillation guided by complex electrograms. Circulation 2007;115:2606–12.
6. Hocini M, Jaïs P, Sanders P, et al. Techniques, evaluation, and consequences of linear block at the left atrial roof in paroxysmal atrial fibrillation: a prospective randomized study. Circulation 2005;112:3688–96.
7. Oral H, Chugh A, Good E, et al. A randomized evaluation of right atrial ablation after left atrial ablation of complex fractionated electrograms for long lasting persistent atrial fibrillation. Circ Arrhythm Electrophysiol 2008;1:6–13.
8. Rostock T, Steven D, Hoffmann B, et al. Chronic atrial fibrillation is a biatrial arrhythmia: data from catheter ablation of chronic atrial fibrillation aiming arrhythmia termination using a sequential ablation approach. Circ Arrhythm Electrophysiol 2008;1:344–53.
9. Jais P, Hocini M, Hsu LF, et al. Technique and results of linear ablation at the mitral isthmus. Circulation 2004;110:2996–3002.
10. Matsuo S, Lim KT, Haissaguerre M. Ablation of chronic atrial fibrillation. Heart Rhythm 2007;4(11):1461–3.
11. O'Neill MD, Wright M, Knecht S, et al. Long-term follow-up of persistent atrial fibrillation ablation using termination as a procedural endpoint. Eur Heart J 2009;30:1105–12.
12. Rostock T, Salukhe TV, Steven D, et al. Long-term single- and multiple-procedure outcome and predictors of success after catheter ablation for persistent atrial fibrillation. Heart Rhythm 2011;8:1391–7.
13. Ammar S, Hessling G, Reents T, et al. Arrhythmia type after persistent atrial fibrillation ablation predicts success of the repeat procedure. Circ Arrhythm Electrophysiol 2011;4:609–14.
14. Jaïs P, Matsuo S, Knecht S, et al. A deductive mapping strategy for atrial tachycardia following atrial fibrillation ablation: importance of localized reentry. J Cardiovasc Electrophysiol 2009;20:480–91.
15. Mohamed U, Skanes AC, Gula LJ, et al. A novel pacing maneuver to localize focal atrial tachycardia. J Cardiovasc Electrophysiol 2007;18:1–6.

Differentiating Right from Left Atrial Tachycardias

Patrizio Pascale, MD*, Ashok J. Shah, MD,
Laurent Roten, MD

KEYWORDS

- Atrial tachycardia • Twelve-lead electrocardiogram • Coronary sinus activation pattern
- Activation and entrainment mapping

KEY POINTS

- The interpretation of the 12-lead electrocardiogram is limited by the reduced voltage and altered activation of the left atrium. The analysis of the surface P wave in the precordial leads may, however, provide clues for a right atrial origin.
- The prevalence of right atrial tachycardias (ATs) after atrial fibrillation ablation is about 10% to 15% and is mainly represented by peritricuspid reentries.
- Analysis of the coronary sinus (CS) activation quickly allows one to rule out a right atrial tachycardia, especially when its activation is different from proximal to distal.
- In the case of proximal to distal CS activation, 23% of ATs are peritricuspid reentries, 4% are focal right atrial ATs, and 73% are located in the left atrium (34% macroreentry and 39% focal).

INTRODUCTION

Mapping of postatrial fibrillation (AF) ablation atrial tachycardias (ATs) is often challenging because multiple foci may coexist and extensive atrial substrate has been targeted. Beyond evident issues of time constraints, a strategy that involves exhaustive activation mapping without a preconceived suspicion of the chamber of interest bears several limitations. First, in the setting of persistent AF ablation, it is often necessary to create multiple activation maps in the event of AT changing during mapping or in case of multiple AT foci or mechanisms. Second, the complexity of mapping often resides in the multiple areas with extensive voltage reduction and/or multiple-component electrograms (EGMs) with altered sequence of activation. In these situations, detailed mapping may prove either difficult or confusing. To rationalize activation and entrainment mapping maneuvers, it is therefore critical for the operator to have a probabilistic clue regarding the chamber of interest, constantly updated after each diagnostic step. This article describes the clues to distinguishing right from left ATs at each of the following step of the diagnostic process:

1. Before starting: initial probability of a right versus left AT
2. Twelve-lead electrocardiogram (ECG) analysis
3. Coronary sinus activation pattern analysis
4. Activation and entrainment mapping

BEFORE STARTING: INITIAL PROBABILITY OF A RIGHT VERSUS LEFT AT

Regardless of the ablation techniques used, ATs occurring after AF ablation most often originate in the left atrium. A precise knowledge of the incidence of right versus left AT after AF ablation is

Conflicts of Interest: None.
Disclosures: None.
Hôpital Cardiologique du Haut-Lévêque, Department of Cardiac Arrhythmias, Université Victor Segalen, Bordeaux II, Bordeaux, France
* Corresponding author. Hôpital Cardiologique du Haut-Lévêque, Department of Cardiac Arrhythmias, Avenue de Magellan, Bordeaux-Pessac 33604, France.
E-mail address: Patrizio.Pascale@chuv.ch

Card Electrophysiol Clin 5 (2013) 169–177
http://dx.doi.org/10.1016/j.ccep.2013.01.009
1877-9182/13/$ – see front matter © 2013 Elsevier Inc. All rights reserved.

essential in implementing a pragmatic mapping strategy. The incidence and type of tachycardia is related to the type of ablation performed during the index procedure. Accordingly, a history of previous linear ablation on the cavotricuspid isthmus (CTI) or of right atrial (RA) EGM-based ablation is expected to influence the probability of AT arising in that chamber. Two successive studies from the authors' group evaluated a total of about 450 ATs that mostly occurred after the stepwise approach for persistent AF, and hence included cases in which biatrial ablation was performed.[1,2] An incidence of 13% of right ATs was observed in both studies. The majority of ATs were CTI-dependent macroreentries (72%). The remaining ATs were centrifugal (27%), either truly focal or localized reentries. Only 1 atypical RA macroreentry was diagnosed. These figures are in line with reports from other groups wherein 10% to 16% of RA ATs were observed after AF

ablation.[3–5] Similarly, CTI-dependent macroreentry represented about three-fourths of those ATs. Despite the fact that all studies included patients in whom RA EGM-guided ablation could be performed, the probability of an RA centrifugal AT remained in the range of 2% while atypical RA macroreentrant ATs were even rarer. Of note, the absence of previous RA ablation does not rule out a centrifugal AT originating in that chamber.[6] Accordingly, even when biatrial ablation has been performed, the AT mapping strategy must take into account the low probability of an RA origin of AT, once a CTI-dependent macroreentry has been ruled out by appropriate activation and entrainment maneuvers.

TWELVE-LEAD ECG ANALYSIS

The characterization of signature P-wave morphology for the ATs occurring after left atrial (LA)

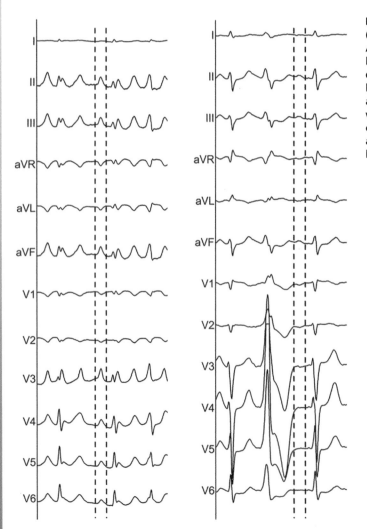

Fig. 1. Twelve-lead electrocardiograms (ECGs) of atrial tachycardia (AT) post-AF ablation with negative P wave in lead V1. (*Left*) A right focal AT was diagnosed successfully and was ablated at the superior base of the right atrial appendage. Note the negative P wave in lead aVL despite a right atrial origin. (*Right*) AT focus successfully ablated at the superior portion of the lateral right atrium.

ablation is much limited by the fact that substrate ablation and/or the creation of lines of block alter the normal activation pattern of the left atrium. Moreover, the LA activation is often either silent or overshadowed by the RA activation because the debulking effect of LA ablation leads to a marked reduction in LA voltage. Chugh and colleagues[7] demonstrated that CTI-dependent reentries occurring after LA ablation for AF often have atypical ECG characteristics. The classic "sawtooth" morphology was not seen in any of the study patients, and 60% of counterclockwise CTI-dependent flutter displayed upright flutter waves in the inferior leads. A negative P wave in left lateral leads (lead I and aVL) has been regarded as a useful sign for distinguishing a left from a right AT.[8,9] However, it has been shown that right focal AT may often lead to negative P waves in lead aVL, especially for foci arising from the crista terminalis.[10,11] Moreover, 60% of CTI-dependent reentries after AF ablation

display a negative P wave in lead aVL.[7] Regarding negative P waves in lead I, they are typically seen in anterolateral LA foci (LA appendage, mitral annulus) or counterclockwise perimitral AT.[9,11,12] However, its use to distinguish right from left AT is again limited by the fact that RA macroreentrant ATs after AF ablation as well as de novo CTI-dependent flutter often display a predominantly negative F wave in lead I.[3,7,13]

However, there are still some features that may distinguish right from left AT in the setting of previous extensive LA ablation. The most useful leads for this purpose are the precordial leads. Two features remain relatively unaffected by altered LA activation or diffuse scarring: the morphology in lead V1 and the "precordial transition." In patients with de novo ATs, a negative P wave in lead V1 has been shown to be highly specific for an RA focal AT.[11] Moreover, in clockwise CTI-dependent flutter, V1 is characterized

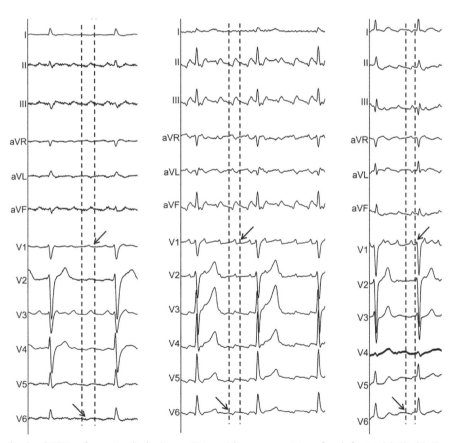

Fig. 2. Twelve-lead ECGs of counterclockwise peritricuspid macroreentries after left atrial (LA) ablation. A classic "sawtooth" morphology in inferior leads is not observed, and evidence of a precordial transition is apparent in all ECGs. Lead V1 demonstrates an upright component (*arrows*). With progression across the precordium, the isoelectric component preceding this upright component becomes negative (by V4 on *left panel*, and V3 on the *middle and right panels*) and the V1 upright component isoelectric. This process produces the overall impression of a positive P wave in V1, which becomes negative by V6 (*arrows*).

by a broad negative P wave in de novo and, to a lesser extent, postablation AT.[7,13] From the authors' experience and the limited data published so far, it appears that a negative P wave in V1 remains a specific marker of a right AT even in patients with previous AF ablation (**Fig. 1**).[3] This finding, however, is rarely observed (about 2% of cases, unpublished data, Pascale et al 2011). In counterclockwise CTI-dependent flutters, lead V1 classically demonstrates an initial isoelectric component followed by an upright component. With progression across the precordium, the initial component rapidly becomes negative and the second component becomes isoelectric usually by V3. This process produces the overall impression of a positive P wave in V1, which becomes negative by V6. In the authors' experience, this precordial transition allows identification of the majority of counterclockwise CTI-dependent flutter presenting with atypical 12-lead ECG after AF ablation, with good specificity (unpublished data; **Fig. 2**). The transition may sometimes be subtle, or a biphasic (negative-positive), rather than negative, deflection may be observed in the left precordial leads. In the study by Chugh and colleagues,[7] evidence of a precordial transition was present in 75% of counterclockwise CTI-dependent flutters arising after AF ablation. Chang and colleagues[3] found that a negative flutter wave

in any of the precordial leads could differentiate a right versus left atrial macroreentrant AT with a 100% specificity. Accordingly, a systematic analysis of the P wave free of T waves should be performed as a first step during mapping. In the absence of the typical sawtooth morphology in the inferior ECG leads, a negative P wave in lead V1 or a precordial transition should prompt RA mapping in cases of consistent coronary sinus (CS) activation pattern.

CS ACTIVATION PATTERN ANALYSIS

As a standard component of the electrophysiologic evaluation, the analysis of the multipolar CS recordings provides a unique opportunity to rapidly guide the operator by disclosing the pattern of activation of the inferior (annular) posterior LA wall. This immediate segmental activation mapping will allow one to rule out an RA origin of the AT in about half of the cases. Based on the analysis of the CS activation pattern in more than 450 ATs after AF ablation, right ATs were always associated with a proximal to distal CS activation; that is, CS bipoles positioned at the CS ostium and lateral CS were, respectively, the earliest and the latest.[1,2] Other CS activation patterns were always associated with an LA origin; these included either a distal to proximal activation, or patterns whereby

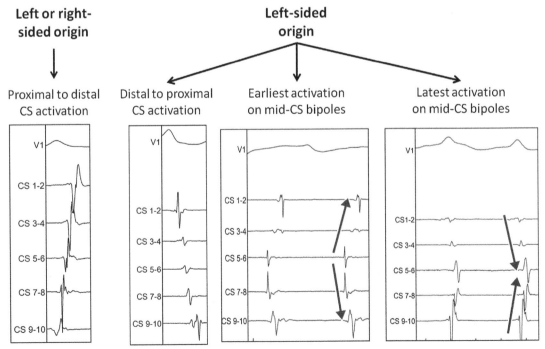

Fig. 3. Sites of origin of post-AF ablation AT according to different coronary sinus (CS) activation patterns observed.

activations recorded on the mid-CS bipoles were either latest or earliest ("chevron" or "fused" patterns, **Fig. 3**). The quick analysis of the CS activation pattern will therefore allow the operator to focus the mapping on the left atrium in about 50% of the cases. Two potential limitations of this approach must, however, be kept in mind. First, though unlikely, the diagnosis of an RA AT, especially CTI-dependent reentry or flutters localized to the superior right atrium, is not formally excluded in cases where the CS is not activated from proximal to distal. Previous reports have shown that CTI-dependent reentries may be associated with a "fused" CS activation pattern whereby the activation of the mid-CS dipoles

are latest (see **Fig. 3**, right panel).[14,15] These cases were related to de novo clockwise peritricuspid AT with the left atrium being predominantly activated over the Bachmann bundle, as opposed to the CS ostium. One should therefore keep in mind this possibility when CS activation is used as a guide to rationalize mapping maneuvers. In the setting of post-AF ablation, previous ablation may delay the conduction through the anterior wall, explaining why this CS activation pattern is seldom observed. Second, a potential drawback of the CS activation pattern lies in the interpretation of sometimes complex EGMs. The authors have previously reported on disparate activation patterns of the LA myocardium and CS

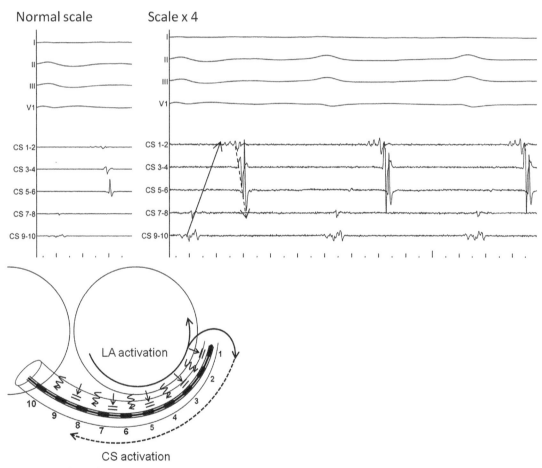

Fig. 4. Recording of disparate LA-CS activation pattern. On normal scale, the CS activation seems to proceed from the lateral to proximal, suggesting a left-sided AT origin. After scale magnification (4 times the usual scale), double potentials become apparent along the whole CS length. The early component consisting of broader and lower-amplitude potentials represents the far-field inferior LA myocardium activity, and demonstrates an activation sequence from proximal to distal (*solid arrow*). The second component, consisting of sharper potentials, represents the activation of the CS musculature itself and propagates in the opposite direction (*dashed arrow*). As illustrated in the lower panel, the activation of the local CS musculature occurs after the activation of the contiguous left atrium when the endocardially propagating wave front crosses over to the distal CS epicardium. Note the long fractionated signals recorded on the most distal bipoles, suggestive of slow conduction at the "turnaround" point of the activation wave front.

musculature as a consequence of partial LA-CS disconnection due to previous ablation performed either endocardially or epicardially (ie, on the inferior left atrium or within the CS, respectively).[16] Because previous ablation and far-field sensing often result in barely discernible signals, the actual sequence of activation of the components that represent the contiguous left atrium is often only apparent after magnifying CS EGMs. Failure to carefully inspect all CS potentials can easily mislead the operator, considering that the more apparent CS muscle activation sequence is in fact opposite to the clinically more relevant LA activation. An example of a misleading distal to proximal CS activation is illustrated in **Fig. 4**. In doubtful cases, endocardial mapping facing the CS should be performed.

Knowledge of the probability of an RA origin once a proximal to distal CS activation has been verified is essential in rationalizing the sequence of diagnostic maneuvers. In 118 consecutive AT post-AF ablations with a proximal to distal CS

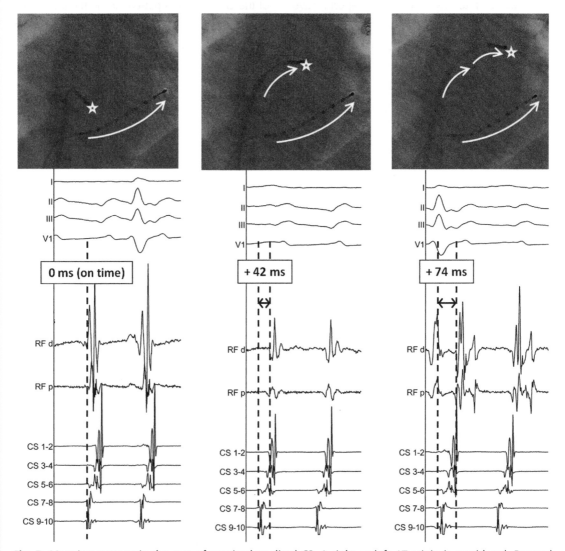

Fig. 5. Mapping strategy in the case of proximal to distal CS. A right or left AT origin is considered. Focused segmental LA mapping starts with the evaluation of the septolateral activation of the (mitral) annular anterior wall. Using CS 9-10 as a reference, and moving the ablation catheter, the local activation time is obtained at the septal, mid, and lateral anterior mitral annulus (*stars*) (0, +42, and +74 milliseconds after the reference, respectively; *dashed lines*). This activation time quickly allows identification of a septal to lateral activation of the anterior annular LA segment, that is, in the same direction as the posterior annular LA activation as depicted by the CS catheter (*white arrows*). A perimitral AT is ruled out. Note that both the anterior and posterior annular segments are activated synchronously, suggesting either a left septal focus or an RA origin. A peritricuspid AT was later diagnosed.

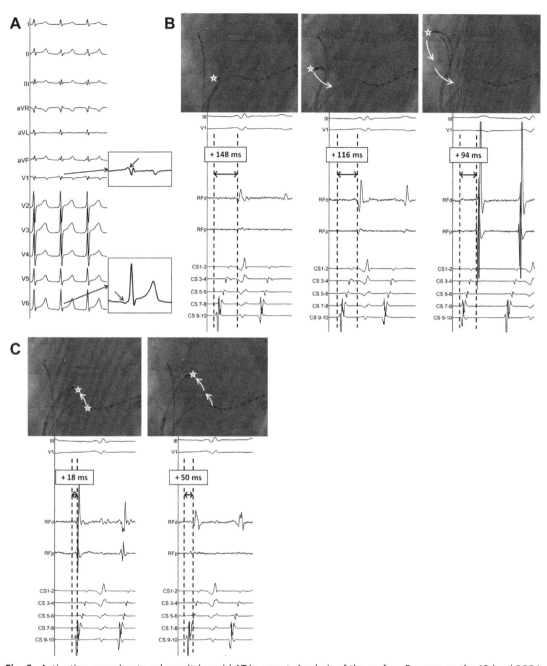

Fig. 6. Activation mapping to rule peritricuspid AT in or out. Analysis of the surface P waves on the 12-lead ECG is limited by the superimposed QRS complexes (*A*). However, a precordial transition is suspected based on an upright component in V1, while a negative (and slightly earlier) P wave is seen in V6 (*arrows*). Mapping of both edges of the cavotricuspid isthmus is therefore performed as a next step. Using CS 9-10 as a reference, and moving the ablation catheter, the local activation time is obtained at the low lateral, lateral, and high lateral tricuspid annulus (*stars*) (+148, +116, and +94 milliseconds after the reference, respectively; *dashed lines*) (*B*). This activation time quickly allows identification of a descending (or lateral to medial) activation of the lateral tricuspid annulus. The septal part of tricuspid annulus is then mapped (*C*). Bipole CS 9-10 is used as a reference and as the timing of the low septal annulus. Moving the ablation catheter, the local activation time is obtained at the mid and anterior septal tricuspid annulus (*stars*) (+18 and +50 milliseconds after the reference, respectively; *dashed lines*). This activation time quickly allows identification of an ascending (or medial to lateral) activation of the septal tricuspid annulus. Note that the cycle length covered by this focused mapping is sequential and spans about 60% of the AT cycle length. A peritricuspid AT is therefore ruled in, later confirmed by 2 entrainment maneuvers on opposite sides of the circuit.

activation, the authors have observed that CTI-dependent reentry represented 23% of cases, with other RA ATs being diagnosed in 4%. Counterclockwise perimitral AT and roof-dependent reentry represented 22% and 12% of cases, respectively, with LA centrifugal ATs representing the remaining 39% of cases.[2] The high probability of a left origin and the substantial proportion of CTI-dependent reentries both imply that the latter diagnosis should be ruled out early in the case of consistent LA activation mapping (ie, septal to lateral anterior mitral annular activation) or, as a first step, in the case of a suggestive 12-lead ECG (see earlier discussion).

ACTIVATION AND ENTRAINMENT MAPPING

As previously discussed, a right AT is considered a plausible differential diagnosis in cases of a proximal to distal CS activation. It is the authors' practice to first concentrate the activation mapping on the left atrium, unless ECG clues favor a right origin or transseptal access is not necessarily foreseen. Atrial activation is mapped by systematically comparing the mapping catheter signals with a reference channel from the decapolar CS catheter (**Fig. 5**). Focused segmental LA mapping is performed, evaluating the "2-axis" activation of both the anterior and posterior wall: the vertical axis activation (ascending or descending wave front) and the septolateral axis activation of its annular segments. The latter should be initially performed because perimitral ATs are more prevalent. A lateral to septal anterior mitral annulus activation (ie, opposite to the CS activation) will rule in perimitral AT, whereas opposite anterior/posterior wall vertical activation will rule in roof-dependent AT. Other activation patterns will rule out both diagnoses. The operator will then either focus the mapping on searching for the earliest activation of an LA centrifugal source or rule out an RA origin in the case of consistent LA mapping, that is, septal to lateral anterior mitral annular activation (see **Fig. 5**). At this stage, RA mapping aims at ruling in or out a CTI-dependent AT. For this purpose either activation or entrainment mapping will be performed. The latter is directly performed in the case of a stable AT. Activation mapping is performed on the CTI and its medial (septum and ostium of the CS) and lateral (tricuspid annulus) edge (**Fig. 6**). Simultaneous activation of both ends of the CTI, double potentials throughout the CTI, or a convergent/colliding activation of both annular sides of the CTI rule out this diagnosis. In the case of a lateral to medial or medial to lateral activation of both tricuspid annulus edges of the CTI, a CTI-dependent AT is ruled in. Further mapping of the anterior tricuspid annulus should be performed to document an activation spanning the full cycle length. To rule out the pitfall of a centrifugal source occurring near a line of previous block (or conduction slowing), entrainment maneuvers on opposite sides of the circuit are mandatory. For this purpose, entrainment is initially performed on the lateral aspect of the CTI, as a good return cycle on the septal side will also occur with several alternative diagnoses. A postpacing interval (PPI) exceeding the AT cycle length by no more than 30 milliseconds on 2 opposite segments of the tricuspid annulus will confirm the diagnosis. A long return cycle on the lateral aspect of the CTI will rule out CTI-dependent AT and further lower the probability of an RA macroreentry or focus. A return cycle less than or equal to 50 milliseconds longer than the AT cycle length will warrant further RA mapping. Otherwise, mapping will concentrate on searching for the earliest activation of a centrifugal source, first in the left atrium then in the right atrium. When the region of interest cannot be located, repeated pacing maneuvers with analysis of the PPI will be used to progressively approach the site of origin of the tachycardia and determine the atrial chamber of interest.[17]

REFERENCES

1. Jais P, Matsuo S, Knecht S, et al. A deductive mapping strategy for atrial tachycardia following atrial fibrillation ablation: importance of localized reentry. J Cardiovasc Electrophysiol 2009;20(5):480–91.
2. Pascale P, Roten L, Shah AJ, et al. Mapping of atrial tachycardia after persistent atrial fibrillation ablation: pattern and timing of the coronary sinus activation as a rapid guidance towards the most likely mechanism. Heart Rhythm 2012;9(5):S266.
3. Chang SL, Tsao HM, Lin YJ, et al. Differentiating macroreentrant from focal atrial tachycardias occurred after circumferential pulmonary vein isolation. J Cardiovasc Electrophysiol 2011;22(7):748–55.
4. Rostock T, Drewitz I, Steven D, et al. Characterization, mapping, and catheter ablation of recurrent atrial tachycardias after stepwise ablation of long-lasting persistent atrial fibrillation. Circ Arrhythm Electrophysiol 2010;3(2):160–9.
5. Tilz RR, Chun KR, Schmidt B, et al. Catheter ablation of long-standing persistent atrial fibrillation: a lesson from circumferential pulmonary vein isolation. J Cardiovasc Electrophysiol 2010;21(10):1085–93.
6. Pappone C, Manguso F, Vicedomini G, et al. Prevention of iatrogenic atrial tachycardia after ablation of atrial fibrillation: a prospective randomized study

comparing circumferential pulmonary vein ablation with a modified approach. Circulation 2004;110(19): 3036–42.

7. Chugh A, Latchamsetty R, Oral H, et al. Characteristics of cavotricuspid isthmus-dependent atrial flutter after left atrial ablation of atrial fibrillation. Circulation 2006;113(5):609–15.

8. Tang CW, Scheinman MM, Van Hare GF, et al. Use of P wave configuration during atrial tachycardia to predict site of origin. J Am Coll Cardiol 1995;26(5): 1315–24.

9. Yamada T, Murakami Y, Yoshida Y, et al. Electrophysiologic and electrocardiographic characteristics and radiofrequency catheter ablation of focal atrial tachycardia originating from the left atrial appendage. Heart Rhythm 2007;4(10):1284–91.

10. Kalman JM, Olgin JE, Karch MR, et al. "Cristal tachycardias": origin of right atrial tachycardias from the crista terminalis identified by intracardiac echocardiography. J Am Coll Cardiol 1998;31(2):451–9.

11. Kistler PM, Roberts-Thomson KC, Haqqani HM, et al. P-wave morphology in focal atrial tachycardia: development of an algorithm to predict the anatomic site of origin. J Am Coll Cardiol 2006;48(5):1010–7.

12. Gerstenfeld EP, Dixit S, Bala R, et al. Surface electrocardiogram characteristics of atrial tachycardias occurring after pulmonary vein isolation. Heart Rhythm 2007;4(9):1136–43.

13. Ndrepepa G, Zrenner B, Deisenhofer I, et al. Relationship between surface electrocardiogram characteristics and endocardial activation sequence in patients with typical atrial flutter. Z Kardiol 2000; 89(6):527–37.

14. Marine JE, Korley VJ, Obioha-Ngwu O, et al. Different patterns of interatrial conduction in clockwise and counterclockwise atrial flutter. Circulation 2001;104(10):1153–7.

15. Oshikawa N, Watanabe I, Masaki R, et al. Relationship between polarity of the flutter wave in the surface ECG and endocardial atrial activation sequence in patients with typical counterclockwise and clockwise atrial flutter. J Interv Card Electrophysiol 2002;7(3):215–23.

16. Pascale P, Shah AJ, Roten L, et al. Disparate activation of the coronary sinus and inferior left atrium during atrial tachycardia after persistent atrial fibrillation ablation: prevalence, pitfalls, and impact on mapping. J Cardiovasc Electrophysiol 2012;23(7): 697–707.

17. Mohamed U, Skanes AC, Gula LJ, et al. A novel pacing maneuver to localize focal atrial tachycardia. J Cardiovasc Electrophysiol 2007;18(1):1–6.

Pulmonary Vein–Associated Tachycardia

Shinsuke Miyazaki, MD*, Ashok J. Shah, MD

KEYWORDS

- Atrial tachycardia • Pulmonary vein • Atrial fibrillation • Catheter ablation

KEY POINTS

- Pulmonary vein (PV)–associated atrial tachycardias (ATs) are commonly observed ATs after atrial fibrillation (AF) ablation.
- Combination of activation and entrainment mapping is required to diagnose the precise mechanism of PV-associated ATs.
- The possibility of PV-associated tachycardia should be considered as the first step in the mapping of ATs after AF ablation; that is, evaluation of PV reconnection is the first step of AT mapping.
- Two types of AT are associated with reconnection after PV isolation: pulmonary vein tachycardia with conduction gap and gap-gap reentrant tachycardia.
- Closing the conduction gap between the PV and the left atrium can eliminate both types of AT completely.

INTRODUCTION

The conduction recovery of a previously ablated pulmonary vein (PV) should be evaluated through appropriate mapping before commencing a systematic deductive diagnostic approach to mapping atrial tachycardia (AT) after atrial fibrillation (AF), which is described elsewhere in this issue. The reason is that the conduction recovery of PVs is associated with recurrence in most paroxysmal and short-lasting persistent AF cases with recurrent atrial tachyarrhythmias. In fact, several authors have shown that reisolation of the PV alone results in a significant improvement in clinical outcome in this subset of patients. Because PV-related tachycardias are completely eliminated through the reisolation of the PV without any additional substrate modification, the precise diagnosis is important. On the contrary, in patients with long-standing persistent AF after extensive AF ablation, the likelihood of AT from PV conduction recovery is much smaller.

A circular mapping catheter helps to evaluate the resumption of PV conduction and identify the site of the conduction gap. Generally, the site of the conduction gap during AT is not difficult to identify because the rhythm is organized, unlike during AF. Recognition of the far-field potential mimicking PV potential is essential during AT and in sinus rhythm.

PV Tachycardia with Conduction Gaps

The AT associated with PV reconnection originates from the muscle sleeve of the reconnected PV. Although prior reports showed that most left ATs after PV isolation had a focal origin from the PV,[1,2] the exact mechanism of these ATs has not been fully evaluated. Gerstenfeld and colleagues[1] reported that the tachycardias typically originated from small areas of preserved voltage on the septal side of the PVs, suggesting small reentrant circuits with a critical isthmus of slow conduction located in isolated areas of PV ostial tissue. Partly

Conflicts of interest: None.
Disclosures: None.
Arrhythmology Department, Hôpital Cardiologique du Haut-Lévêque and the Université Victor Segalen Bordeaux II, Avenue de Magellan, Bordeaux, Pessac Cedex 33604, France
* Corresponding author. Hôpital Haut Lévêque, Bordeaux-Pessac 33604, France.
E-mail address: mshinsuke@k3.dion.ne.jp

Card Electrophysiol Clin 5 (2013) 179–187
http://dx.doi.org/10.1016/j.ccep.2013.01.011
1877-9182/13/$ – see front matter © 2013 Elsevier Inc. All rights reserved.

cardiacEP.theclinics.com

ablated myocardium can create slow conduction and unidirectional block necessary to support reentry, whereas uncoupled segments of myocardium from prior ablation may create the substrate for automatic or triggered arrhythmias. Shah and colleagues[3] reported localized reentrant AT with discrete, narrow, and unique zones of marked slow conduction at or in the vicinity of previously ablated PV ostial sites. Marked slow conduction and an adjacent anatomic defect played a critical role in stabilizing these small circuits. Moving the circular mapping catheter systematically to each PV ostium and searching for mid-diastolic or fractionated potential often can suggest a critical area of the reentrant circuit. These types of ATs show centrifugal activation pattern from the source.

Sometimes, confined PV fibrillation/tachycardia results in recurrent atrial tachyarrhythmias via reconnection after PV antrum isolation. The left atrial activation occurs 1-to-1 or with Wenckebach conduction through the gap in the circumferential PV lesion-set. Because the conduction gaps between the left atrium and the PV are limited, the type of recurrence (AF or AT) depends on the conduction property of the gap (**Figs. 1–4**). **Fig. 5** shows an example of a bystander PV tachycardia confined to the PV in a patient with previously ablated longstanding AF.[4] During AT mapping, PV tachycardia with a cycle length of 180 ms was recorded in the left superior PV, with seemingly 4 to 3 conduction patterns between the PV and the LA. However, the termination of this tachycardia did not have any impact on the clinical AT, which suggested its bystander role.

Gap-Gap Reentrant Tachycardia

LA-PV reentrant tachycardia is observed in patients with arrhythmia recurrence associated with PV reconnection.[5,6] This tachycardia is an iatrogenic reentry using multiple gaps between the LA and the PV. The following diagnostic criteria were proposed previously[5]: (1) recovered PV conduction with one-to-one LA-PV or PV-LA conduction during tachycardia; (2) identification of sites with perfect entrainment within the PVs and the LA near the involved PVs; (3) entrainment within the PVs with identical P-wave morphology as during tachycardia; (4) identification of 2 conduction gaps in the previous circumferential lesion set: 1 conduction gap presents as the entrance site with earliest PV activation and 1 as the exit with earliest atrial activation; and (5) termination of the tachycardia through radiofrequency delivery at either the entrance or the exit site. **Figs. 6–10** show a typical case of gap-gap reentry after ipsilateral circumferential PV isolation, wherein the activation mapping of recurrent AT demonstrated

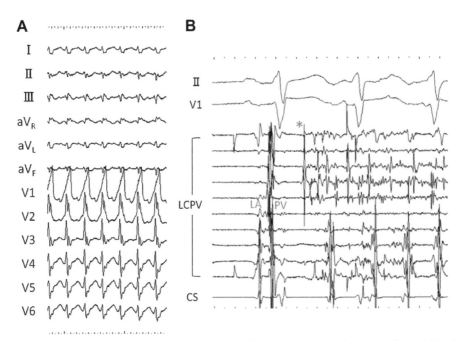

Fig. 1. Case 1. (*A*) A 12-lead electrogram of the recurrent clinical AT arising after circumferential ipsilateral PV isolation. (*B*) A circular mapping catheter is placed in the LCPV. The mapping catheter shows the conduction recovery and the initiation of clinical AT from the LCPV (*asterisk*). CS, coronary sinus; LA, left atrial potential; LCPV, left common pulmonary vein; PV, pulmonary vein potential.

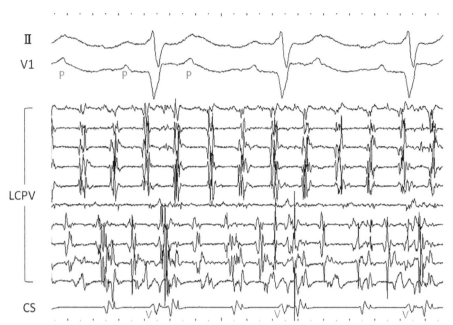

Fig. 2. Case 1. A circular mapping catheter is placed in LCPV. During the clinical AT, PV tachycardia/fibrillation is observed in the LCPV. Note the P wave morphology on surface electrocardiogram. CS, coronary sinus; LCPV, left common pulmonary vein; P, P wave; V, ventricular potential.

a reentrant pattern and the entrainment mapping showed that the right PVs and the LA septum were the integral parts of the tachycardia circuit. Exiting the PV from near the roof of the right superior vein, the activation spread to the LA septum anteriorly and reentered the PV via a gap in the circumferential lesion at the bottom of the right inferior vein, wherefrom the electroanatomic continuity between the 2 PVs effected the wavefront's return to the right superior vein (see **Fig. 6**, dotted

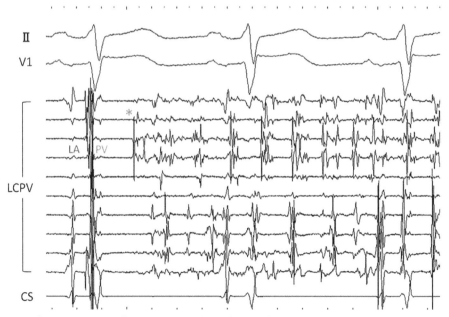

Fig. 3. Case 1. After restoration of sinus rhythm through radiofrequency application, confined PV fibrillation (*asterisk*) is observed in the LCPV. Note that exit block is evident, but not the entrance block. CS, coronary sinus; LA, left atrial potential; LCPV, left common pulmonary vein; PV, pulmonary vein potential; V, ventricular potential.

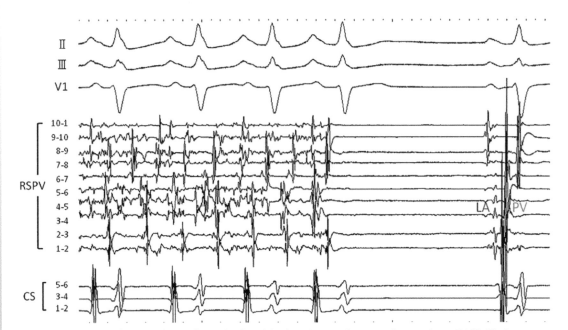

Fig. 4. Case 2. A circular mapping catheter is placed in the RSPV at the second procedure. PV fibrillation causes clinical AT, which terminated with cessation of PV firing. CS, coronary sinus; LA, left atrial potential; PV, pulmonary vein potential; RSPV, right superior pulmonary vein. (*Adapted from* Miyazaki S, Kobori A, Komatsu Y, et al. Clinical implication of adenosine test at repeat atrial fibrillation ablation procedure: the importance of detecting dormant thoracic vein conduction. Circ Arrhythm Electrophysiol 2012;5:1117–23; with permission.)

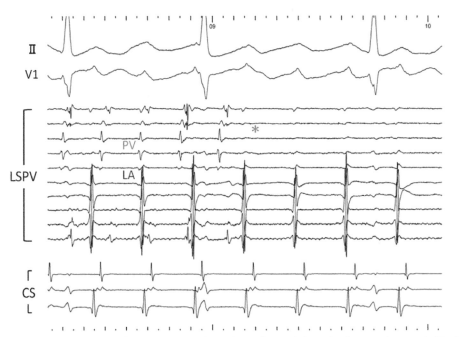

Fig. 5. Case 3. During clinical AT, pulmonary vein tachycardia with a cycle length of 180 ms is recorded in the LSPV, with possibly 4 to 3 conduction patterns between the pulmonary vein and the left atrium. However, the termination of this tachycardia (*asterisk*) does not have any impact on the clinical AT, which suggests that it was a bystander pulmonary vein tachycardia. CS, coronary sinus; LA, left atrial potential; LSPV, left superior PV; PV, pulmonary vein potential; V, ventricular potential. (*Adapted from* Miyazaki S, Taniguchi H, Iesaka Y. Pulmonary vein tachycardia during atrial tachycardia in the context of atrial fibrillation ablation. Europace 2012;14:1; with permission.)

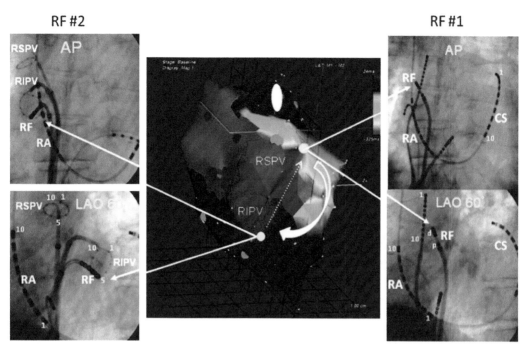

Fig. 6. Case 4. A 3-dimensional activation map of AT also showing 2 conduction gaps between the LA and right ipsilateral PVs. White arrows indicate the activation sequence of the tachycardia. The right panel shows the roof of right superior PV ostium where AT was terminated by a radiofrequency application, and the left panel shows the bottom of right inferior PV ostium where ipsilateral right PVs were isolated again by spot radiofrequency application. AP, anteroposterior view; d, distal; LAO, left oblique view; p, proximal; RA, right atrium; RF, radiofrequency ablation catheter; RIPV, right inferior PV; RSPV, right superior pulmonary vein. (*Adapted from* Miyazaki S, Shah AJ, Kobori A, et al. How to approach reentrant atrial tachycardia after atrial fibrillation ablation. Circ Arrhythm Electrophysiol 2012;5:e1–7; with permission.)

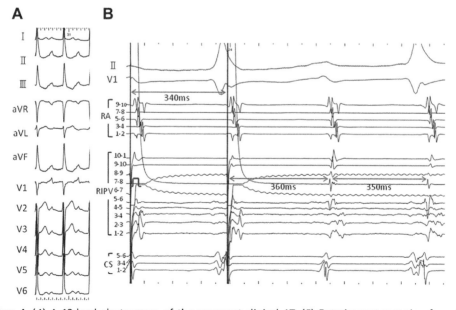

Fig. 7. Case 4. (*A*) A 12-lead electrogram of the recurrent clinical AT. (*B*) Entrainment mapping from the RIPV shows that ΔPPI-TCL was 10 ms. CS, coronary sinus; PPI, postpacing interval; RA, right atrium; RIPV, right inferior PV; TCL, tachycardia cycle length; V, ventricular potential. (*Adapted from* Miyazaki S, Shah AJ, Kobori A, et al. How to approach reentrant atrial tachycardia after atrial fibrillation ablation. Circ Arrhythm Electrophysiol 2012;5:e1–7; with permission.)

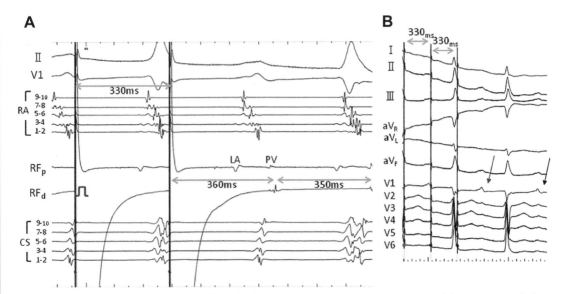

Fig. 8. Case 4. (*A*) Entrainment mapping from the RSPV showed that ΔPPI-TCL was 10 ms. (*B*) P-wave morphology during RSPV entrainment (*red arrow*) is identical to that observed during tachycardia (*blue arrow*). CS, coronary sinus; LA, left atrial potential; PPI, postpacing interval; PV, pulmonary vein potential; RA, right atrium; RF, radiofrequency ablation catheter; TCL, tachycardia cycle length; V, ventricular potential. (*Adapted from* Miyazaki S, Shah AJ, Kobori A, et al. How to approach reentrant atrial tachycardia after atrial fibrillation ablation. Circ Arrhythm Electrophysiol 2012;5:e1–7; with permission.)

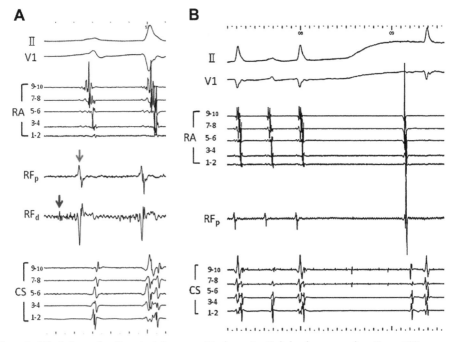

Fig. 9. Case 4. (*A*) A long fractionated low-amplitude potential (*red arrow*; duration: 140 ms, amplitude: 0.044 mV) is recorded on the roof of the RSPV ostium during AT. Note that atrial potential is observed on the proximal mapping catheter (*blue arrow*). (*B*) Gap-gap reentrant tachycardia is terminated after 4.5 seconds of radiofrequency application at this site. CS, coronary sinus; RA, right atrium; RF, radiofrequency ablation catheter; RSPV, right superior pulmonary vein; V, ventricular potential. (*Adapted from* Miyazaki S, Shah AJ, Kobori A, et al. How to approach reentrant atrial tachycardia after atrial fibrillation ablation. Circ Arrhythm Electrophysiol 2012;5:e1–7; with permission.)

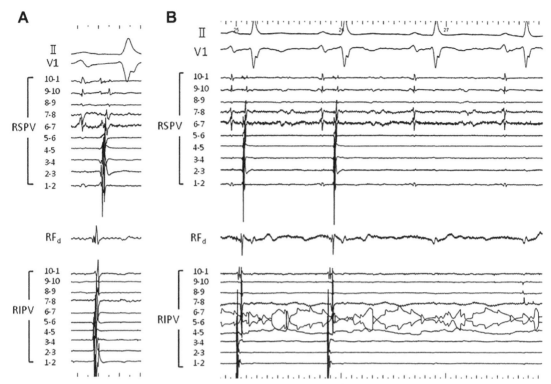

Fig. 10. Case 4. (*A*) An ablation catheter was placed at the bottom of RIPV ostium in sinus rhythm. (*B*) RSPV was activated after RIPV in sinus rhythm. The earliest potential on the circular mapping catheter was recorded at the bottom of the RIPV (bipole 5-6). Ipsilateral right PVs were simultaneously isolated after 4.2 seconds of radiofrequency application at this site. RF, radiofrequency ablation catheter; RIPV, right inferior PV; RSPV, right superior pulmonary vein. (*Adapted from* Miyazaki S, Shah AJ, Kobori A, et al. How to approach reentrant atrial tachycardia after atrial fibrillation ablation. Circ Arrhythm Electrophysiol 2012;5:e1–7; with permission.)

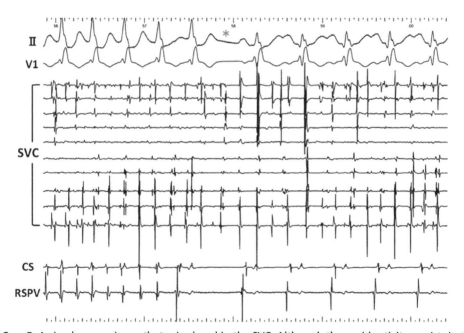

Fig. 11. Case 5. A circular mapping catheter is placed in the SVC. Although the rapid activity persists in the SVC, AT converts to sinus rhythm (*asterisk*) during radiofrequency application at the atriocaval junction. CS, coronary sinus; RSPV, right superior pulmonary vein; SVC, superior vena cava; V, ventricular potential. (*Adapted from* Miyazaki S, Kuwahara T, Takahashi A. Confined driver of atrial fibrillation in the superior vena cava. J Cardiovasc Electrophysiol 2012;23:440; with permission.)

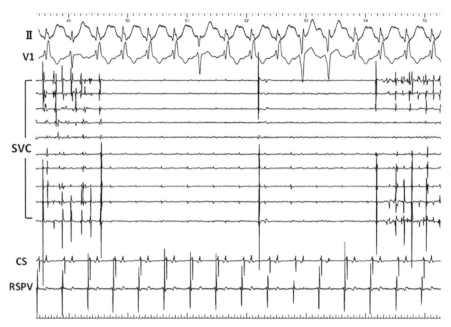

Fig. 12. Case 5. After spontaneous and transient termination of the rapid activity, dissociated activity was observed in the SVC during sinus rhythm, which suggested bidirectional electrical conduction block (also considering findings seen in **Fig. 11**) between the SVC and the right atrium. CS, coronary sinus; RSPV, right superior pulmonary vein; SVC, superior vena cava; V, ventricular potential. (*Adapted from* Miyazaki S, Kuwahara T, Takahashi A. Confined driver of atrial fibrillation in the superior vena cava. J Cardiovasc Electrophysiol 2012;23:440; with permission.)

arrow). The gap between right superior vein and the LA was the site of critical isthmus with slow conduction. The first radiofrequency delivery at that site immediately terminated the tachycardia (see **Fig. 9**). The second radiofrequency delivery, at the bottom of right inferior vein now in sinus rhythm, simultaneously isolated the right PVs from the LA (see **Fig. 10**), confirming that the 2 veins were mutually connected and the conduction gap in right inferior vein was critical for reentry of the tachycardia wavefront from LA into the PVs. These findings confirm that the mechanism of this AT was LA-PV reentry, with active involvement of 2 gaps in the previously deployed circumferential ablation line. This tachycardia could have been potentially misdiagnosed as focal AT arising from the right PVs in the absence of entrainment mapping. This type of AT could involve even a single PV if segmental PV isolation is performed previously.

Superior Vena Cava–Associated Tachycardia

The superior vena cava (SVC) can be the source of AT after AF ablation. Myocardial extension to the SVC with associated arrhythmogenic activity has been demonstrated previously. SVC has been recognized as one of the important sources of triggers that initiate and also drive AF. Because the

connection between the SVC and the right atrium is less intense than the PV-LA connection, SVC fibrillation/tachycardia not rarely presents AT. **Fig. 11** shows a clinical example of SVC fibrillation.[7] During radiofrequency application, AT/AF converted to sinus rhythm despite persistent rapid activity in the SVC, suggesting an exit block from the SVC to the right atrium. A few minutes later, the rapid activity in the SVC terminated spontaneously and transiently only to be replaced by slow dissociated activity (**Fig. 12**), which now suggests an entrance block from the right atrium to the SVC.

SUMMARY

PV-associated ATs are commonly observed after AF ablation. Assessment of PV isolation is the important first step in mapping these ATs. The combination of activation and entrainment mapping is required to reach the precise diagnosis.

REFERENCES

1. Gerstenfeld EP, Callans DJ, Dixit S, et al. Mechanisms of organized left atrial tachycardias occurring after pulmonary vein isolation. Circulation 2004;110:1351–7.
2. Ouyang F, Antz M, Ernst S, et al. Recovered pulmonary vein conduction as a dominant factor for recurrent

atrial tachyarrhythmias after complete circular isolation of the pulmonary veins: lessons from double Lasso technique. Circulation 2005;111:127–35.

3. Shah D, Sunthorn H, Burri H, et al. Narrow, slow-conducting isthmus dependent left atrial reentry developing after ablation for atrial fibrillation: ECG characterisation and elimination by focal RF ablation. J Cardiovasc Electrophysiol 2006;17:508–15.

4. Miyazaki S, Taniguchi H, Iesaka Y. Pulmonary vein tachycardia during atrial tachycardia in the context of atrial fibrillation ablation. Europace 2012;14:1.

5. Satomi K, Bänsch D, Tilz R, et al. Left atrial and pulmonary vein macroreentrant tachycardia associated with double conduction gaps: a novel type of man-made tachycardia after circumferential pulmonary vein isolation. Heart Rhythm 2008;5:43–51.

6. Miyazaki S, Shah AJ, Kobori A, et al. How to approach reentrant atrial tachycardia after atrial fibrillation ablation. Circ Arrhythm Electrophysiol 2012;5:e1–7.

7. Miyazaki S, Kuwahara T, Takahashi A. Confined driver of atrial fibrillation in the superior vena cava. J Cardiovasc Electrophysiol 2012;23:440.

Diagnosis of Macroreentrant Atrial Tachycardia

Laurent Roten, MD[a],*, Patrizio Pascale, MD[b]

KEYWORDS

- Atrial tachycardia • Macroreentry • Catheter ablation

KEY POINTS

- Half of the atrial tachycardia cases after persistent atrial fibrillation ablation are macroreentry, commonly called atrial "flutter."
- In clinical practice 3 macroreentrant atrial tachycardias demarcated by major anatomic structures are encountered, by far: atrial tachycardia rotating around the mitral annulus, the ipsilateral pulmonary venous lesion through the roof, and the tricuspid orifice.
- Because the tachycardia circuit is well defined, mapping a few points along the circuit to check if they are sequentially activated can quickly allow the assessment of macroreentry.
- If the activation pattern is compatible with macroreentry, further mapping requires confirmation by entrainment mapping.

INTRODUCTION

Termination of atrial fibrillation (AF) to atrial tachycardia (AT) is frequently observed during AF ablation, especially when substrate ablation is performed. The stepwise ablation approach even aims at terminating AF to either AT or sinus rhythm and most patients are terminated to AT rather than sinus rhythm.[1] In the case of AF termination during the index procedure, arrhythmia is more likely to recur in the form of AT.[2] Finally, if linear ablation is attempted but not successful, arrhythmia often recurs in the form of AT and any successfully ablated line that recovers will also promote AT.[3] For these reasons, AT are very common during or after persistent AF ablation. To succeed in ablation of AT, its mechanism must be identified and the tachycardia circuit or origin must be mapped. In almost half of the cases, the mechanism of AT following AF ablation is macroreentry.[4] This article describes the strategy to map macroreentrant AT without using a 3-dimensional mapping system and the following article elsewhere in this issue exemplifies it.

ATRIAL TACHYCARDIA—BASICS RECAPITULATED

An AT is defined as an organized atrial rhythm with a stable morphology and a stable activation sequence in both atria. The latter can easily be verified by analyzing the relation of signals recorded by 2 catheters placed in both atria. The cycle length of an AT is usually stable, although there may be some variation depending on the underlying mechanism (see later discussion). The 2 following types of AT can be clearly differentiated based on their electrophysiologic mechanisms[5]:

- Focal AT (due to an automatic, triggered, or microreentrant mechanism)
- Macroreentrant AT (including typical atrial flutter and other well-characterized macroreentrant circuits)

First, tachycardia cycle length variability should be analyzed (**Fig. 1**). If it exceeds 15% of tachycardia cycle length, a focal mechanism can be

---

Conflict of Interest: None.

[a] Department of Cardiology, Inselspital, Bern University Hospital, University of Bern, Freiburgstrasse, Bern 3010, Switzerland; [b] Department of Cardiology, Centre Hospitalier Universitaire Vaudois et Université de Lausanne, Rue du Bugnon 21, Lausanne 1011, Switzerland
* Corresponding author.
E-mail address: laurent.roten@insel.ch

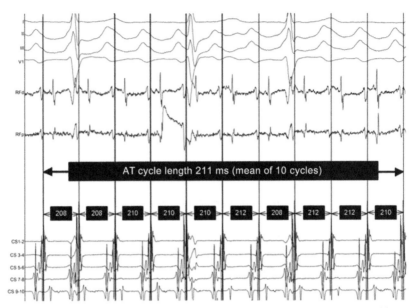

Fig. 1. The assessment of cycle length variability. Mean tachycardia cycle length is measured by averaging 10 or more tachycardia cycle lengths. The cycle length variability is calculated by dividing the difference between the longest and shortest tachycardia cycle length by the mean tachycardia cycle length. In this example, tachycardia cycle length variability is $(212 - 208)/211 = 0.019 = 2\%$.

suspected.[4] Mapping of focal AT is described in more detail in the article, "Diagnosis of Focal-Source Atrial Tachycardia" of this issue. If tachycardia cycle length variability is less than 15%, both a macroreentrant and a focal mechanism are possible. In such a case, a macroreentrant tachycardia should first be ruled in or out because it is easier to investigate it than a focal tachycardia.

Basically, there are only 3 possibilities for a macroreentrant AT following AF ablation:

- Mitral isthmus-dependent AT (perimitral AT)
- Roof-dependent AT
- Cavotricuspid isthmus-dependent AT (typical and reverse typical atrial flutter)

For each of these 3 AT, activation can propagate 1 way or the other around the anatomic obstacle: around the mitral annulus for mitral isthmus-dependent AT and around the tricuspid annulus for cavotricuspid isthmus-dependent AT. For roof-dependent AT, the activation revolves around the left or the right pulmonary veins or both with the roof forming the critical isthmus. To complicate matters, a combination of perimitral and roof-dependent AT (double loop) can also be present or an AT circuit can alternate between 2 gaps on the same isthmus. These AT may present with cycle length alterations.

Activation Mapping

Activation mapping is the first step in the diagnostic pursuit of any macroreentrant AT. A decapolar catheter positioned in the coronary sinus is most useful for 2 reasons: first, coronary sinus activation is always evident and a change in activation pattern is immediately recognized; second, a catheter in the coronary sinus is very stable and can be used as a reference for activation mapping performed by another roving catheter in the atria.

By mapping different atrial segments relative to a reference signal in the coronary sinus, a simple activation map can be quickly generated. Such an activation map need not be very detailed but should just help decipher the global activation patterns. In the left atrium, it suffices to map whether the direction of activation is low to high or opposite on the posterior and anterior walls and whether it is septal to lateral or opposite on the inferior and anterior walls. In the right atrium, the direction of activation around the tricuspid annulus should primarily be mapped. With this information, it can easily be concluded whether a macroreentrant tachycardia is possible, in which case this has to be confirmed by entrainment maneuvers. If a macroreentrant AT is already ruled out by activation mapping, a focal AT should be investigated.

Entrainment Mapping

Entrainment mapping is the second step in the diagnostic pursuit of AT. It is the confirmatory step for establishing the diagnosis of macroreentry. The aim is to verify active participation of the respective atrial segments in the presumed tachycardia circuit. Entrainment is performed by pacing from distinct atrial segments at a cycle length 20 ms less than tachycardia cycle length. Before assessing postpacing intervals, successful global tachycardia entrainment should be confirmed based on general principles of entrainment.[6] To delineate the tachycardia, circuit entrainment should be performed from 3 different atrial segments of the presumed tachycardia circuit. If all postpacing intervals in these segments are within 30 ms of the tachycardia cycle length, the postulated macroreentry is confirmed and the focal tachycardia is ruled out.

PERIMITRAL AT
Activation Mapping

Perimitral AT can propagate either clockwise or counterclockwise around the mitral annulus when viewed from the apex of the heart (**Fig. 2**). The activation patterns of the coronary sinus and the anterosuperior part of the mitral annulus define the direction of propagation of perimitral AT.

Activation mapping in clockwise perimitral AT
- Coronary sinus activation: distal to proximal
- Anterosuperior part of the mitral annulus: septal to lateral

Activation mapping in counter-clockwise perimitral AT
- Coronary sinus activation: proximal to distal
- Anterosuperior part of the mitral annulus: lateral to septal

In both clockwise and counterclockwise perimitral AT, the posterior and anterior left atrial walls are activated from inferior to superior. If the coronary sinus has previously been ablated, its activation has to be analyzed with caution as one can be misled by a partially disconnected coronary sinus.[7] In case of any doubt, the left atrial inferior wall activation relative to coronary sinus activation should be verified with the roving catheter.

Entrainment Mapping

Tachycardia entrainment should be performed from 3 different atrial segments around the mitral annulus (**Fig. 3**). Sites that present distinct, high-amplitude signals should always be preferred. Typical sites to confirm a perimitral AT by entrainment mapping are the proximal and distal coronary sinus (unless the coronary sinus is partially disconnected), the anteroseptal, anterolateral, and lateral left atrium. If extensive ablation has previously been performed on the mitral isthmus, postpacing intervals may exceed tachycardia cycle length by more than 30 ms at segments of the mitral isthmus that are remote from the gap site. If such a situation is suspected, entrainment should be repeated from different segments of the mitral isthmus.

ROOF-DEPENDENT ATRIAL TACHYCARDIA
Activation Mapping

Roof-dependent AT can propagate clockwise or counterclockwise around the right or the left pulmonary veins or simultaneously around both the right and the left pulmonary veins (**Fig. 4**). Characteristically, the activation of the posterior and the anterior wall of the left atrium occurs in opposite directions. Activation of the coronary sinus is nonspecific but often shows a chevron (<) or inverse chevron (>) pattern when the

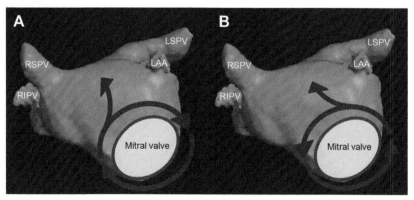

Fig. 2. Clockwise (*A*) and counterclockwise (*B*) perimitral AT. Note that the anterior wall is activated from low to high (inferior to superior) in both cases. LAA, left atrial appendage; LSPV, left superior pulmonary vein; RIPV, right inferior pulmonary vein; RSPV, right superior pulmonary vein.

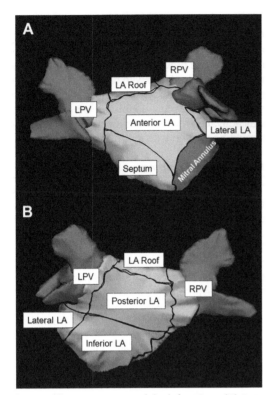

Fig. 3. Different segments of the left atrium. (*A*) Anterior view; (*B*) Posterior view. LA, left atrium; LPV, left pulmonary veins; RPV, right pulmonary veins.

posterior left atrial wall is activated from high to low or low to high, respectively.

High to low posterior left atrial activation
- Anterior left atrial wall will be activated from low to high

- Coronary sinus activation may show a chevron pattern

Low to high posterior left atrial activation
- Anterior left atrial wall will be activated from high to low
- Coronary sinus activation may show an inverse chevron pattern

Entrainment Mapping

To confirm a roof-dependent AT, entrainment can be performed from the low and high posterior and anterior left atrial wall. Depending on whether the tachycardia revolves around the left or right pulmonary veins, postpacing intervals will exceed tachycardia cycle length by more than 30 ms when entrainment is performed on the anterior septum or anterolateral left atrium, respectively. As with perimitral AT, postpacing intervals will also exceed tachycardia cycle length by more than 30 ms in cases with previous ablation along the roof line, depending on the location of the gap site and entrainment; for example, if the gap site is located close to the right pulmonary veins, entrainment close to the left pulmonary veins may result in longer postpacing intervals and vice versa.

PERITRICUSPID ATRIAL TACHYCARDIA

Cavotricuspid isthmus-dependent AT is the least common type of macroreentrant AT encountered during or after persistent AF ablation.[4] A 12-lead electrocardiogram (ECG) may show the typical morphology of cavotricuspid isthmus-dependent AT. However, after extensive left atrial ablation, the reliability of the 12-lead ECG in diagnosing

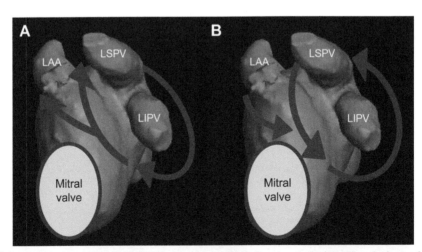

Fig. 4. Roof-dependent AT with tachycardia circuit around the left pulmonary veins in a clockwise fashion (*A*) or counter-clockwise fashion (*B*) when viewed from the left lateral side. Note that impulse conduction can proceed between either LSPV and LAA, LAA and mitral annulus, or both (this is also the case for perimitral AT). LAA, left atrial appendage; LIPV, left inferior pulmonary vein; LSPV, left superior pulmonary vein.

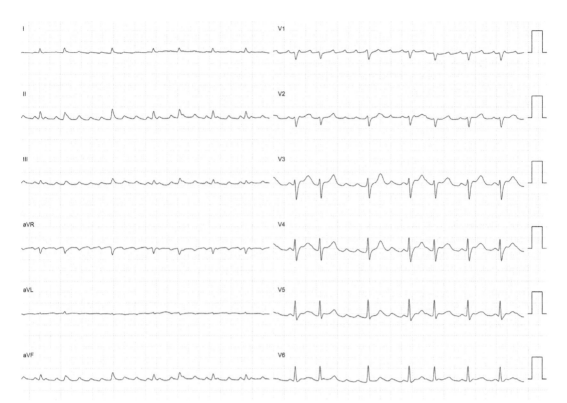

Fig. 5. Macroreentrant AT occurring in a patient after pulmonary vein isolation and extensive left atrial ablation. The flutter waves are positive in the inferior leads and in leads V1-V6, which is not the typical ECG morphology of cavotricuspid isthmus-dependent AT. However, this AT was cavotricuspid isthmus-dependent and ablation at that site terminated it.

cavotricuspid isthmus-dependent AT is severely impaired, as exemplified by **Fig. 5**. Standard activation and entrainment mapping should therefore be performed to rule in or out cavotricuspid isthmus-dependent AT irrespective of the morphology of the flutter waves on the 12-lead ECG.

Activation Mapping

Contrary to perimitral and roof-dependent AT, the entire tachycardia circuit can be mapped within the right atrium in cavotricuspid isthmus-dependent AT and the left atrium is activated as a bystander only. On the left atrium, both the coronary sinus and the anterior wall are activated from septal to lateral unless previous ablation has severely impaired conduction at these segments.

Entrainment Mapping

The usual sites for entrainment to confirm cavotricuspid isthmus-dependent AT are the lateral right atrium, the right atrial septum, and the cavotricuspid isthmus. It has recently been demonstrated that postpacing intervals may exceed tachycardia cycle length by more than 30 ms, depending on the entrainment site, pacing cycle length, and tachycardia cycle length variability.[8] Although the cavotricuspid isthmus necessarily forms part of the tachycardia circuit, there is significant variation of the path of the circuit in the superior part of the right atrium.[9] These facts need to be considered when analyzing the results of entrainment mapping.

SUMMARY

AT is frequent after persistent AF ablation and about half of them are macroreentrant AT. Three different macroreentrant tachycardias may be encountered in these patients: perimitral AT, roof-dependent AT, and cavotricuspid isthmus-dependent AT. The tachycardia circuit can be rapidly assessed by a decapolar catheter in the coronary sinus and additional activation mapping. Once the tachycardia circuit has been mapped, active participation of 3 of its segments should be proven by entrainment mapping to confirm macroreentry.

REFERENCES

1. Haissaguerre M, Sanders P, Hocini M, et al. Catheter ablation of long-lasting persistent atrial fibrillation: critical structures for termination. J Cardiovasc Electrophysiol 2005;16:1125–37.
2. O'Neill MD, Wright M, Knecht S, et al. Long-term follow-up of persistent atrial fibrillation ablation using termination as a procedural endpoint. Eur Heart J 2009;30:1105–12.
3. Knecht S, Hocini M, Wright M, et al. Left atrial linear lesions are required for successful treatment of persistent atrial fibrillation. Eur Heart J 2008;29: 2359–66.
4. Jais P, Matsuo S, Knecht S, et al. A deductive mapping strategy for atrial tachycardia following atrial fibrillation ablation: importance of localized reentry. J Cardiovasc Electrophysiol 2009;20:480–91.
5. Saoudi N, Cosio F, Waldo A, et al. A classification of atrial flutter and regular atrial tachycardia according to electrophysiological mechanisms and anatomical bases; a Statement from a Joint Expert Group from the Working Group of Arrhythmias of the European Society of Cardiology and the North American Society of Pacing and Electrophysiology. Eur Heart J 2001;22: 1162–82.
6. Cosio FG, Lopez Gil M, Arribas F, et al. Mechanisms of entrainment of human common flutter studied with multiple endocardial recordings. Circulation 1994;89:2117–25.
7. Pascale P, Shah AJ, Roten L, et al. Disparate activation of the coronary sinus and inferior left atrium during atrial tachycardia after persistent atrial fibrillation ablation: prevalence, pitfalls, and impact on mapping. J Cardiovasc Electrophysiol 2012;23: 697–707.
8. Vollmann D, Stevenson WG, Luthje L, et al. Misleading long post-pacing interval after entrainment of typical atrial flutter from the cavotricuspid isthmus. J Am Coll Cardiol 2012;59:819–24.
9. Santucci PA, Varma N, Cytron J, et al. Electroanatomic mapping of postpacing intervals clarifies the complete active circuit and variants in atrial flutter. Heart Rhythm 2009;6:1586–95.

Typical Examples of Macroreentrant Atrial Tachycardia

Laurent Roten, MD[a],*, Patrizio Pascale, MD[b]

KEYWORDS

- Atrial tachycardia • Macroreentry • Catheter ablation

KEY POINTS

- Macroreentrant atrial tachycardia can be mapped without the use of a 3-dimensional mapping system.
- Three different macroreentrant atrial tachycardias are generally encountered and mapping of these is illustrated in 3 cases.

CASE 1

A 61-year-old woman complains of palpitations. A 12-lead electrocardiogram (ECG) shows typical atrial flutter (**Fig. 1**) and an ablation procedure is scheduled. A quadripolar catheter is introduced into the coronary sinus (CS 1–2; CS 3–4) and an ablation catheter is placed at the cavotricuspid isthmus (ABL 1–2; ABL 3–4). Tachycardia cycle length (mean of 10 cycles) is 233 ms and tachycardia cycle length variability 9% ([246–225]/233 = 0.09 (**Fig. 2**). There is a stable relation between the coronary sinus and the cavotricuspid isthmus (see **Fig. 2**, red arrows). Next, activation around the tricuspid annulus is mapped: the ablation catheter is moved around the tricuspid annulus and the local delay relative to a reference signal in the proximal CS (CS 1–2) is measured (**Fig. 3**). Relative to the reference signal, activation is delayed on the mid septum by 26 ms (see **Fig. 3**A), on the roof by 64 ms (see **Fig. 3**B), on the lateral right atrium by 144 ms (see **Fig. 3**C), and on the cavotricuspid isthmus by 196 ms (see **Fig. 3**D). Therefore, activation proceeds around the tricuspid annulus in a counterclockwise (see **Fig. 3**, red arrows) direction, compatible with

typical atrial flutter. Next, the tachycardia is entrained at 4 different sites of the presumed tachycardia circuit by burst pacing with a cycle length of 200 ms (**Fig. 4**). The 4 entrainment sites in **Fig. 4** correspond to the sites shown in **Fig. 3** (A, mid septal; B, roof; C, lateral right atrium; D, cavotricuspid isthmus). The postpacing interval is within 30 ms of the tachycardia cycle length at all 4 sites, thereby confirming that the tachycardia is counterclockwise cavotricuspid isthmus-dependent typical atrial flutter. Ablation of the cavotricuspid isthmus terminates the tachycardia to sinus rhythm (not shown).

CASE 2

A 55-year-old man is referred for atrial tachycardia (AT) ablation. He has had 2 previous ablation procedures for persistent atrial fibrillation. **Fig. 5** shows the 12-lead ECG of the AT. The morphology of the flutter waves is stable. A decapolar catheter is introduced into the coronary sinus (CS 1–2; CS 3–4; CS 5–6; CS 7–8; CS 9–10) and an ablation catheter (RF d [distal radiofrequency ablation catheter]; RF p [proximal radiofrequency ablation catheter]) is placed on the His bundle. There is a stable

Conflict of Interest: None.
[a] Department of Cardiology, Inselspital, Bern University Hospital, University of Bern, Freiburgstrasse, Bern 3010, Switzerland; [b] Department of Cardiology, Centre Hospitalier Universitaire Vaudois et Université de Lausanne, Rue du Bugnon 21, Lausanne 1011, Switzerland
* Corresponding author.
E-mail address: laurent.roten@insel.ch

Card Electrophysiol Clin 5 (2013) 195–206
http://dx.doi.org/10.1016/j.ccep.2013.01.013
1877-9182/13/$ – see front matter © 2013 Elsevier Inc. All rights reserved

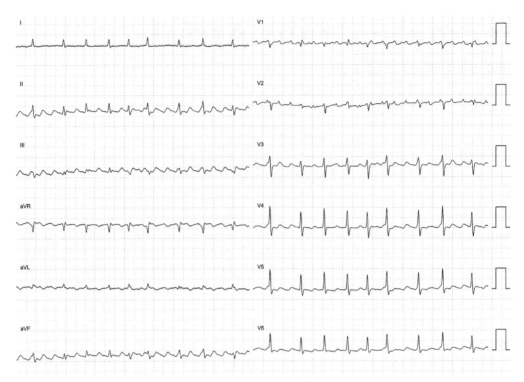

Fig. 1. In the patient in case 1, 12-lead ECG shows typical atrial flutter.

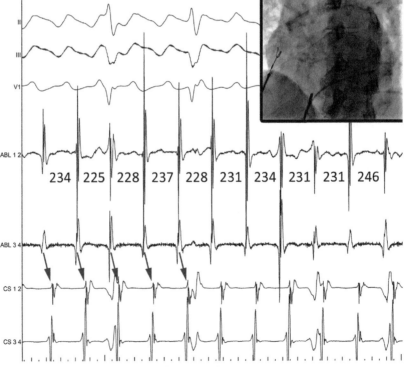

Fig. 2. Tachycardia cycle length. See text for explanation of arrows.

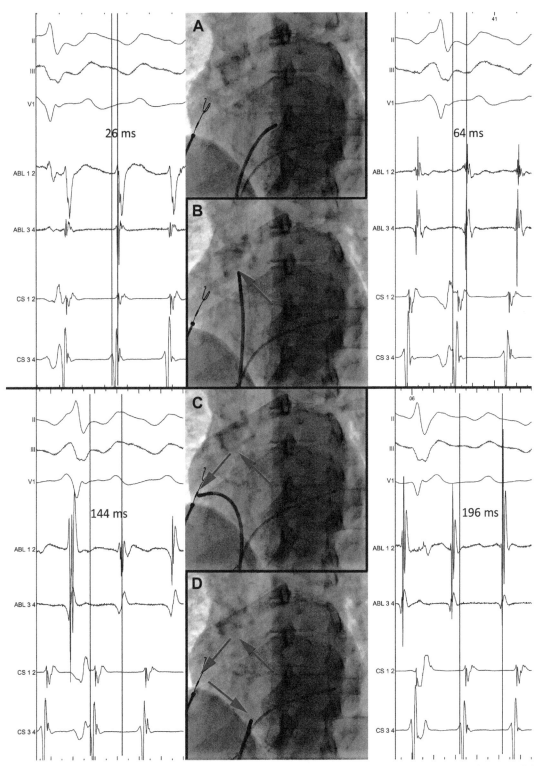

Fig. 3. Mapping of activation around the tricuspid annulus. Activation is delayed on the mid septum by 26 ms (*A*), on the roof by 64 ms (*B*), on the lateral right atrium by 144 ms (*C*), and on the cavotricuspid isthmus by 196 ms (*D*). See text for explanation of arrows.

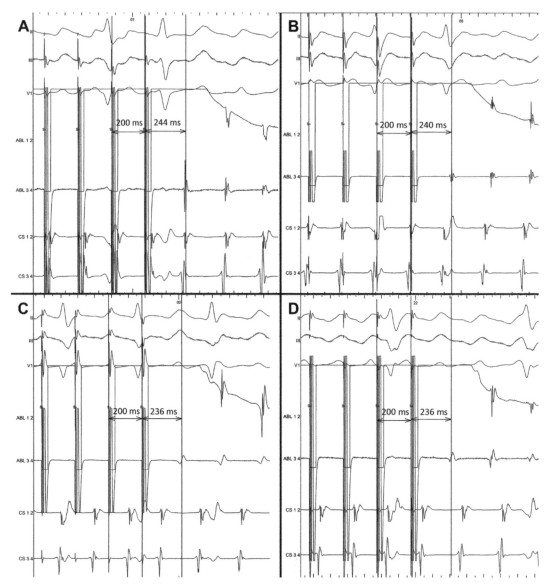

Fig. 4. Four entrainment sites correspond to the sites shown in **Fig. 3** (*A*, mid septal; *B*, roof; *C*, lateral right atrium; *D*, cavotricuspid isthmus).

relation between activation of the left (CS catheter) and right atria (RF catheter) as evidenced in **Fig. 6**. Tachycardia cycle length calculated as the mean of 10 cycles is 218 ms. Tachycardia cycle length variability is 10% ([232–210]/218 = 0.10) and therefore both a macro-reentrant and a focal mechanism are possible. Activation of the coronary sinus is from distal to proximal bipoles (**Fig. 6**, red arrows). Next, activation mapping is performed relative to a reference signal on the coronary sinus catheter (in this case, CS 1–2). The roving catheter is placed on the low posterior left atrial wall (**Fig. 7A**), where double potentials can be recorded. The second potential is 60 ms after the reference signal. Then the roving catheter is displaced toward the high

posterior left atrial wall (see **Fig. 7B**). There, the potentials are further delayed relative to the reference signal (90 ms later). Thus, the posterior left atrial wall is activated from low to high (green star and arrow in **Fig. 7B**). Similarly, the anterior left atrial wall is mapped. First, the catheter is placed on the high anterior left atrial wall (see **Fig. 7C**), where the signal follows the reference signal by 140 ms. Then, the roving catheter is moved lower on the anterior left atrial wall where the signal is further delayed (170 ms; see **Fig. 7D**). Therefore, the anterior left atrial wall is activated from high to low (green star and arrow in **Fig. 7D**) and activation mapping of the posterior and anterior left atrial wall is compatible with a roof-dependent AT.

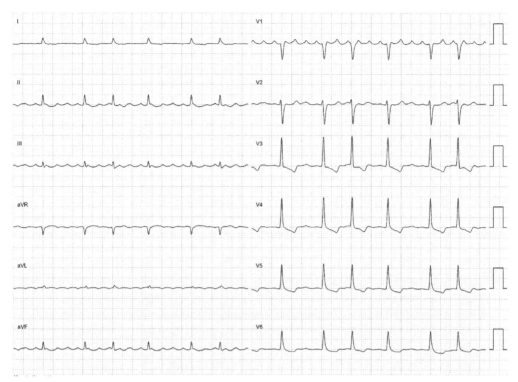

Fig. 5. 12-Lead ECG of the AT in the patient in case 2.

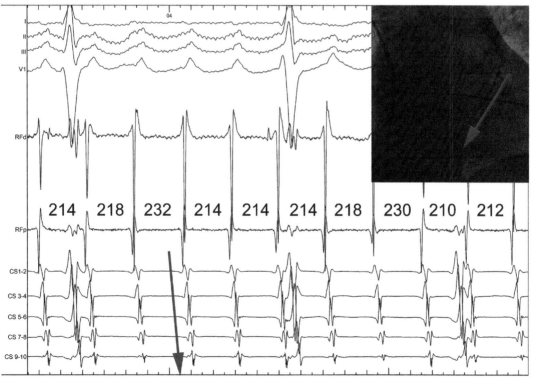

Fig. 6. Stable relation between activation of the left (CS catheter) and right atria (RF catheter). See text for explanation of arrows.

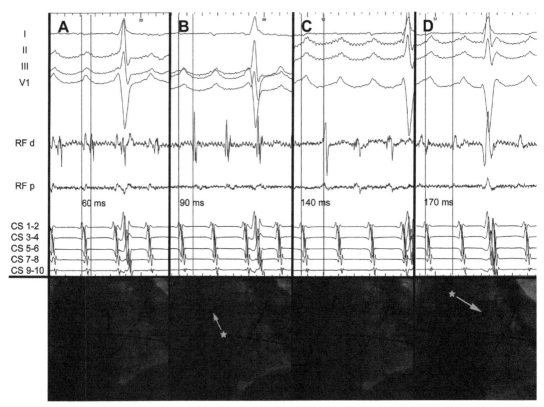

Fig. 7. (A) Roving catheter placed on the low posterior left atrial wall. (B) Roving catheter displaced toward the high posterior left atrial wall. There the potentials are further delayed relative to the reference signal (90 ms later). Thus, the posterior left atrial wall is activated from low to high (*green arrow*). (C) The catheter is placed on the high anterior left atrial wall where the signal follows the reference signal by 140 ms. (D) The roving catheter is moved lower on the anterior left atrial wall where the signal is further delayed. Therefore, the anterior left atrial wall is activated from high to low (*green arrow*).

As a last (confirmatory) step, the tachycardia is entrained with a pacing cycle length of 200 ms from different segments of the presumed tachycardia circuit: from the lateral anterior left atrial wall (**Fig. 8**A, B), from the high posterior left atrial wall (see **Fig. 8**C, D), and from the low posterior left atrial wall (not shown). Entrainment is successful from these sites as evidenced by an acceleration of the cycle length in the coronary sinus to the pacing cycle length (**Fig. 8**A, C). Postpacing intervals are within 30 ms of the tachycardia cycle length of 218 ms at all the sites (240 ms and 230 ms, respectively, for the sites shown). This confirms that the tachycardia mechanism is a roof-dependent macroreentry. Ablation of the roof line terminates AT to sinus rhythm.

CASE 3

A 55-year-old patient underwent stepwise catheter ablation of persistent atrial fibrillation. Two years later he developed an AT (**Fig. 9**) and a second procedure was performed. A decapolar catheter in the coronary sinus (CS 1–2; CS 3–4; CS 5–6; CS 7–8; CS 9–10) showed proximal to distal CS activation (red arrows, **Fig. 10**). Tachycardia cycle length calculated as the mean of 10 cycles was 210 ms (see **Fig. 10**). Tachycardia cycle length variability was 3% ([214–208]/210 = 0.03). Activation mapping was performed relative to a reference signal in CS 1–2. First, the posterior left atrial wall was mapped: on the low posterior left atrial wall activation was delayed by 176 ms (**Fig. 11**A) and on the high posterior left atrial wall activation was delayed by 190 ms relative to CS 1–2 (see **Fig. 11**B). The posterior left atrial wall therefore was activated from low to high (see **Fig. 11**B, red arrow). Next, the activation of the anterior left atrial wall was examined: on the low anterior left atrial wall activation was delayed by 68 ms (see **Fig. 11**C) and on the high anterior left atrial wall activation was delayed by 76 ms relative to the reference signal (see **Fig. 11**D). Thus, the anterior left atrial wall was also activated from low to high

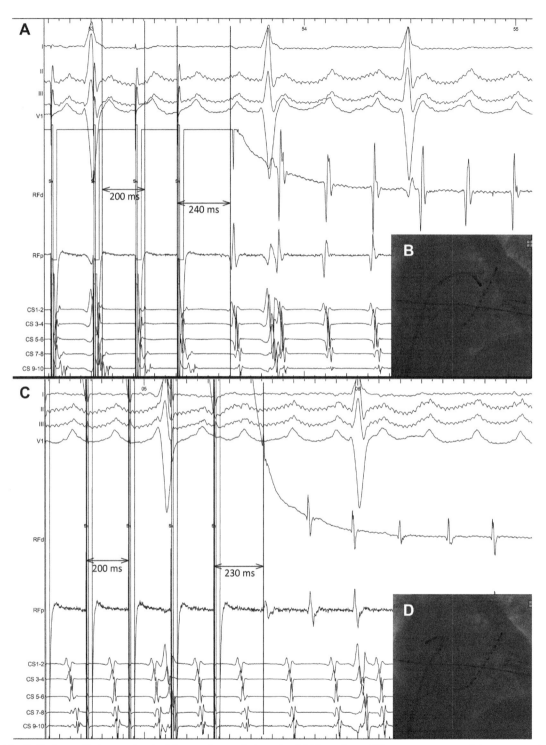

Fig. 8. Tachycardia is entrained with a pacing cycle length of 200 ms from different segments of the presumed tachycardia circuit: from the lateral anterior left atrial wall (A, B), from the high posterior left atrial wall (C, D), and from the low posterior left atrial wall (not shown).

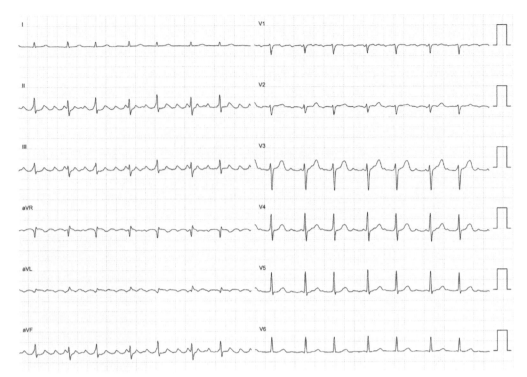

Fig. 9. AT in the patient in case 3.

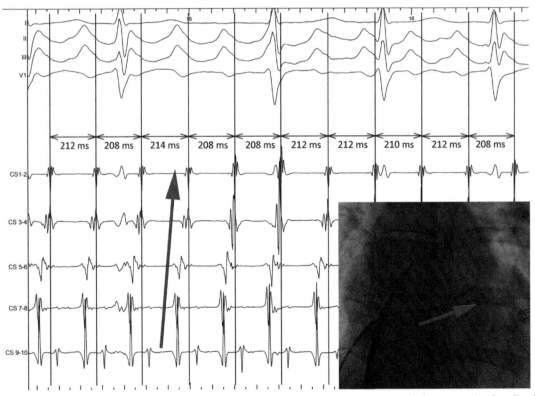

Fig. 10. Decapolar catheter in the coronary sinus (CS 1–2; CS 3–4; CS 5–6; CS 7–8; CS 9–10) shown proximal to distal CS activation. See text for explanation of arrows.

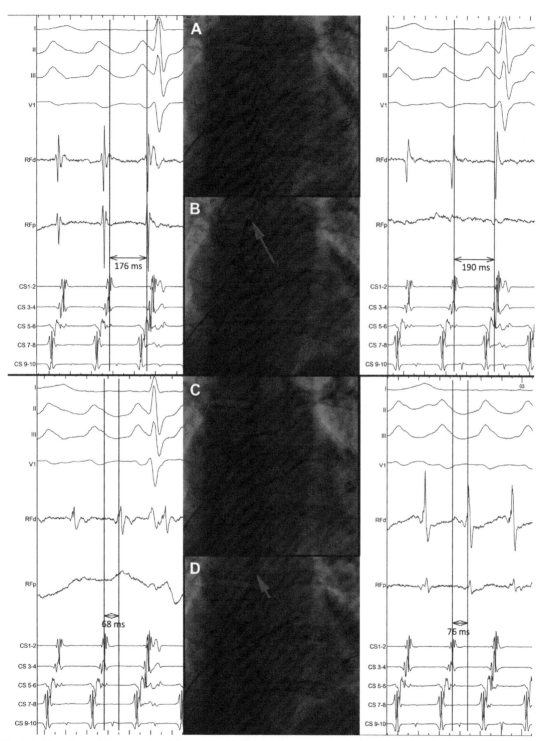

Fig. 11. Mapping of the posterior left atrial wall. On the low posterior left atrial wall activation was delayed by 176 ms (*A*) and on the high posterior left atrial wall activation was delayed by 190 ms relative to CS 1–2 (*B*). The posterior left atrial wall therefore was activated from low to high (*red arrow*). Next, the activation of the anterior left atrial wall was examined: on the low anterior left atrial wall activation was delayed by 68 ms (*C*) and on the high anterior left atrial wall activation was delayed by 76 ms relative to the reference signal (*D*).

(see **Fig. 11**D, red arrow) ruling out a roof-dependent atrial tachycardia. The roving catheter then was placed on the lateral (**Fig. 12**A), mid (see **Fig. 12**B), and septal (see **Fig. 12**C) anterior left atrial walls where the signal was delayed by 42 ms, 64 ms, and 118 ms, respectively, relative to the reference signal. Therefore, the anterior left atrial wall was activated from lateral to septal (see **Fig. 12**C, red arrows) and because the inferior-posterior wall was activated from septal to lateral (according to the coronary sinus catheter), activation mapping was compatible with a counterclockwise perimitral AT. Finally, the tachycardia was entrained at a cycle length of 200 ms from the posterolateral left atrial wall (see **Fig. 12**A), the mid anterior left atrial wall (see **Fig. 12**B), and the

proximal CS (not shown). During entrainment, the cycle length in the coronary sinus accelerated to the entrainment cycle length of 200 ms (see **Fig. 13**A, B). The postpacing intervals were within 30 ms of the tachycardia cycle length at both the posterolateral left atrial wall (238 ms) and the mid anterior left atrial wall (216 ms), which confirmed the activation mapping-based diagnosis of perimitral AT. The mitral isthmus is ablated. Because endocardial ablation was not successful, an epicardial ablation from within the coronary sinus was performed, where double potentials were recorded (**Fig. 14**A, B). During ablation the catheter was slowly pulled back to the position shown in **Fig. 14**C, where the AT terminates to sinus rhythm (see **Fig. 14**D).

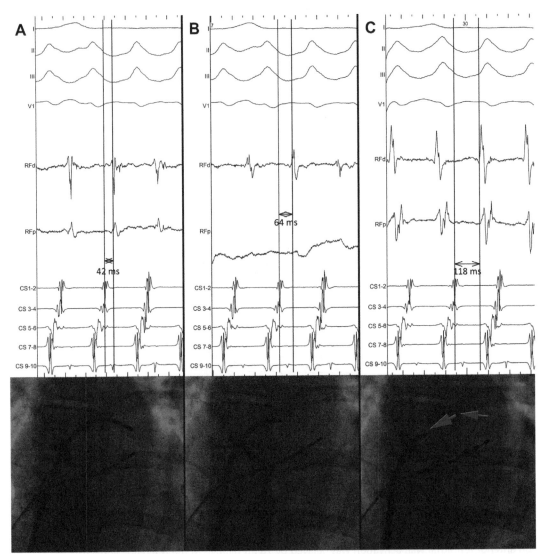

Fig. 12. Roving catheter placed on the lateral (*A*), mid (*B*), and septal (*C*) anterior left atrial walls where the signal was delayed by 42 ms, 64 ms, and 118 ms, respectively, relative to the reference signal. Red arrows in C show that the anterior left atrial wall was activated from lateral to septal.

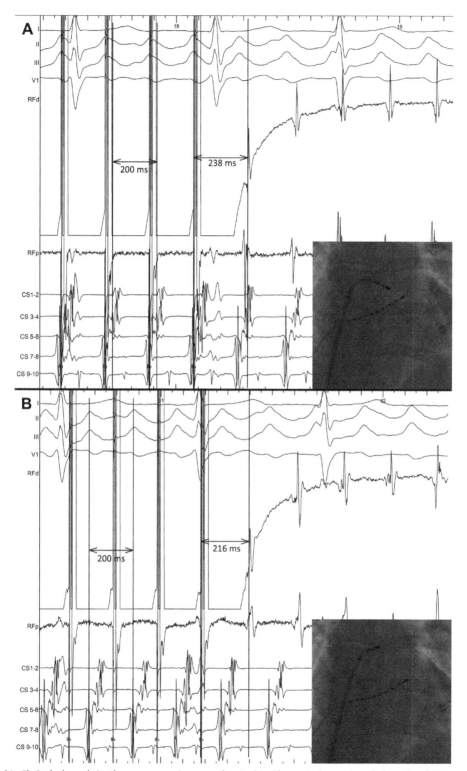

Fig. 13. (*A, B*) Cycle length in the coronary sinus accelerated to the entrainment cycle length of 200 ms.

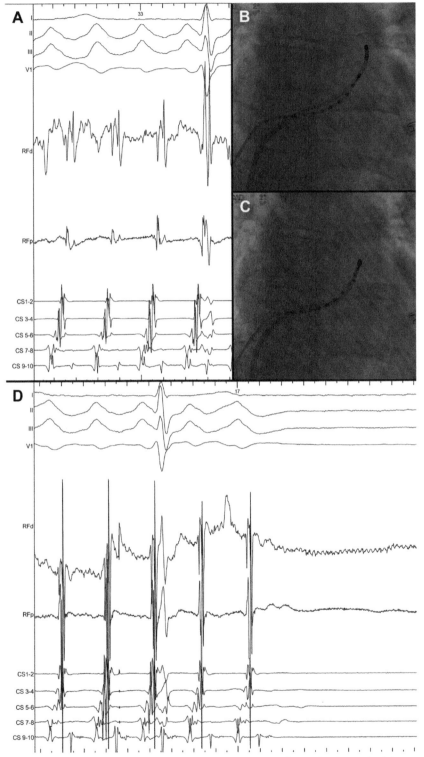

Fig. 14. Epicardial ablation from within the coronary sinus was performed, where double potentials were recorded (*A, B*). During ablation, the catheter was slowly pulled back to the position shown in (*C*), where the AT terminated to sinus rhythm (*D*).

Diagnosis of Focal-Source Atrial Tachycardia
Localized Reentry and Focal Atrial Tachycardia

Michala Pedersen, MD*, Ashok J. Shah, MD,
Patrizio Pascale, MD, Meleze Hocini, MD

KEYWORDS

• Atrial tachycardia • Focal source • Local reentry • Mapping • Activation • Entrainment

KEY POINTS

• The foundation of diagnosing focal-source atrial tachycardia (AT) is activation mapping.
• Once macro reentrant tachycardias have been ruled out, the art is to gently move around, small distances at a time, to map the direction of activation of the tachycardia.
• Once the source of activation causing a centrifugal spread has been localized, entrainment mapping on the spot of origin is used to confirm the diagnosis.
• Focal and localized reentry ATs usually require discrete ablation at a critical spot.

INTRODUCTION

Focal-source atrial tachycardias (ATs) are common after atrial fibrillation (AF) ablation, accounting for 25% to 54% of all post-AF ablation ATs in different series.[1–4] Among these, localized reentry is the most common AT mechanism, in 1 study representing 74% of focal-source ATs.[1] Focal-source and localized reentry ATs usually require discrete ablation at a critical spot.[1,2]

Fig. 1 depicts these mechanisms.

Focal tachycardia is defined as centrifugal activation originating from a discrete site that incorporates automaticity, triggered activity, and reentrant mechanisms, where less than 75% of the cycle can be mapped in the region of interest.

Localized reentry is a type of focal-source AT wherein the tachycardia circuit, usually about 2 cm in diameter, involves 1 or 2 adjacent segments such that more than 70% of the cycle length lies within 1 segment. The remainder of the atria is activated centrifugally.

PREFERENTIAL REGIONS OF FOCAL-SOURCE AT

The preferential regions for focal-source AT are the pulmonary venous ostia, the left septum, and the mouth of the left atrial appendage (**Fig. 2**).

ATs are often related to ablation sites from earlier targeted areas during circumferential pulmonary vein isolation and electrogram-based AF ablation.

Conflicts of Interest: None.
Disclosures: None.
Department of Electrophysiology, Hôpital Cardiologique du Haut-Lévêque, Université Victor Segalen Bordeaux II, Bordeaux, Pessac 33604, France.
* Corresponding author. Hôpital Haut Lévêque, Bordeaux, Pessac 33604, France.
E-mail address: michalapedersen@doctors.org.uk

Card Electrophysiol Clin 5 (2013) 207–214
http://dx.doi.org/10.1016/j.ccep.2013.01.006
1877-9182/13/$ – see front matter © 2013 Elsevier Inc. All rights reserved.

cardiacEP.theclinics.com

FOCAL   LOCALIZED REENTRY

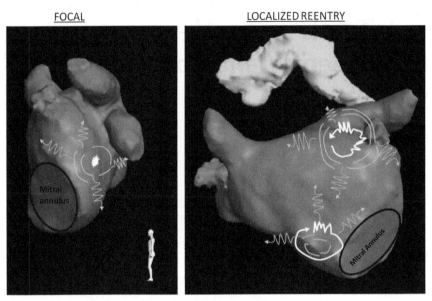

Fig. 1. Mechanisms of focal and localized reentry atrial tachycardias.

The presence of pre-existing left atrial scar (which may be idiopathic or related to underlying structural heart disease) may also result in local slow conduction areas, predisposing to localized reentry.

Injury or edema of the atrial tissue provoked by radiofrequency applications could cause the substrate for arrhythmia by creating an anchoring point potentially able to maintain reentry within the local region. Therefore the mechanism of AT

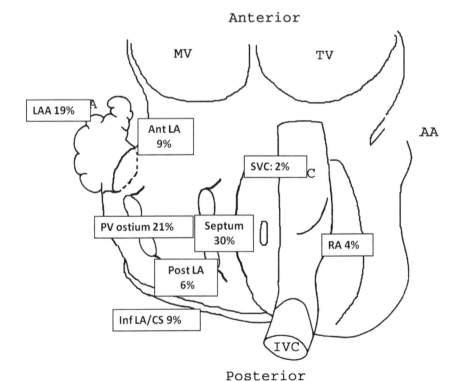

Fig. 2. Preferential regions of focal-source atrial tachycardias. LAA, left atrial appendage; Ant LA, anterior LA; Post LA, posterior LA; Inf LA/CS, inferior left atrium/coronary sinus; PV ostium, pulmonary vein ostium; SVC, superior vena cava; IVC, inferior vena cava; RA, right atrium; MV, mitral valve; TV, tricuspid valve.

after AF ablation may be different than that of spontaneous AT.

MAPPING FOCAL SOURCE ATS

As a rule of thumb, while macro reentrant AT is easy to diagnose but difficult to treat, focal-source and localized reentrant ATs are difficult to map but easy to ablate.

As described in the article by Dr Miyazaki in this issue, the first step in the diagnostic pursuit of any AT is assessment of the stability of the AT cycle length (CL).

Unstable ATs (ATCL variation >15%) are usually focal-source or localized reentrant ATs, and most are unlikely to be macro reentrant ATs. On the other hand, stable ATs could be due to any of these 3 types.

For a stable AT, it is always easier to rule out macro reentry than the remaining types.

Once it is established that the tachycardia is not any of the 3 types of macro reentry (described by Dr Roten in this issue), activation and entrainment mapping are undertaken to localize the focal-source AT.

ACTIVATION MAPPING

Activation mapping is the first step in the diagnostic pursuit of any stable AT. It must be followed by entrainment mapping to establish the final diagnosis.

Activation mapping can be undertaken using a decapolar catheter positioned in the coronary sinus (CS) and an ablation catheter introduced through the sheath into the left atrium.

Left atrial activation is determined before the right. The activation of the anterior and posterior walls is assessed superior-inferior and septal-laterally. This, together with entrainment mapping, will rule out a macro reentrant tachycardia and will home in on the anatomic origin of the AT.

The atrial activation pattern reflects the direction of centrifugal propagation of AT from the focal source. In a single tachycardia cycle, the activation pattern of CS (proximal to distal or distal to proximal or simultaneously none) and the left atrial activation pattern, which do not conform to macro reentrant mechanism, provide a useful guide to localizing the source.

Once known whether the centrifugal activation is from anterior or posterior, or superior or inferior, gently move the catheter in this area and compare the activation time to a fixed electrogram. The beginning of the P-wave is ideal as a fixed reference, but if no clear upstroke any other atrial signal can be used, ideally the earliest signal, often the earliest CS signal, is ideal. Move the catheter until

the very earliest point is located. This can take some perseverance.

A fragmented electrogram spanning over 50% to 75% of the tachycardia cycle length is suggestive of the site of localized reentrant circuit. If it spans less than 50%, it is likely to be a focal AT. However, the 2 types cannot always be distinguished.

Example of Activation Mapping

After ruling out the 3 macroreentrant ATs, localization of the source of focal AT with ATCL 320 milliseconds was undertaken. CS activation occurred from proximal-to-distal direction, suggestive of septal-to-lateral activation of the posterior left atrial wall. Anteriorly, the left atrial activation was determined to be in the septal-to-lateral direction.

As shown in **Fig. 3**, the site of earliest activation was then determined to a fixed reference at the earliest bipole on the decapolar catheter (ie, CS 9–10). The site A was 74 milliseconds earlier than the reference. The local activation of sites B and C was progressively earlier than site A. The local activation of site D was the earliest (204 milliseconds earlier than the reference).

CONFIRMATION OF SOURCE BY ENTRAINMENT MAPPING

Although the site of earliest activation is localized based on activation mapping, the site being the source should be ascertained with the tachycardia entrainment maneuvers.

During entrainment of the focal tachycardia, analysis of the postpacing interval (PPI) can also be used to progressively approach the site of origin of the tachycardia as described by Mohamed and colleagues.[5] A PPI less than or equal to 30 milliseconds is considered as indicative of the proximity of the pacing site to the tachycardia source. In the presence of PPI exceeding the cycle length more than 50 milliseconds, entrainment should be performed from another segment of the atrium.

Conversely to the characteristics of macro reentry, PPI less than or equal to 30 milliseconds cannot be found in more than 1 atrial segment for focal AT. In other words, the atrial segment with PPI less than or equal to 30 milliseconds harbors the source of focal AT.

Example of Entrainment Mapping

Fig. 4 shows the entrainment mapping following the activation mapping shown in **Fig. 3**.

PPI-ATCL at the site of earliest local activation (site D) was more than 100 milliseconds, ruling out site D as the source of AT.

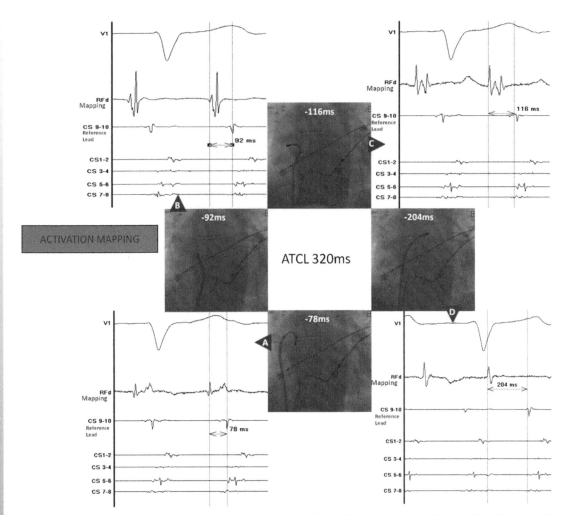

Fig. 3. Activation mapping of focal source atrial tachycardies. Each of parts A, B, C and D show the ablation catheter 'homing in' on the earliest activation as compared to the reference lead. The site A was 74 milliseconds earlier than the reference. The local activation of sites B and was progressively earlier than site A. The local activation of site D was the earliest.

The PPI got shorter while moving from site A to site B, suggestive of a more proximal location of site B to the tachycardia focus than site A.

Continued mapping in and around site B yielded site C with earlier local activation (-116 milliseconds) and PPI less than 30 milliseconds. Site C was therefore the source of focal tachycardia.

AT was terminated successfully during ablation at site C.

MAPPING USING MULTIELECTRODE CATHETERS

An aid in determining left atrial areas/zones for ablation is the use of multipolar catheters, such as the LASSO catheter or the PENTA-RAY

catheter (Thermocool 3.5 mm tip catheter, Biosense Webster Inc, Diamond Bar, California), with 10 and 20 poles, respectively. The advantage, apart from the high density of electrograms, is the temporal and directional information such closely organized catheter poles can provide. These catheters can prove particularly useful in mapping focal and localized reentrant tachycardias, as will be shown in the example.

Example of Mapping Using MultiElectrode Catheters

Fig. 5 shows a 12-lead electrocardiogram of an AT with ATCL of 220 seconds and a cycle length variation of less than 5%.

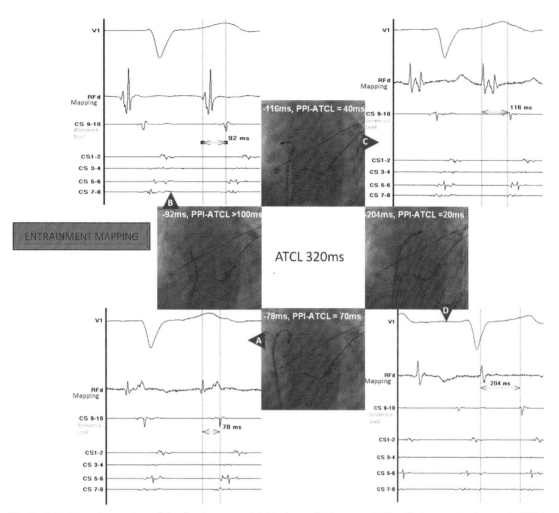

Fig. 4. Entrainment mapping of the focal-source atrial tachycardia (same as in **Fig. 3**). Post pacing intervals (PPI) is shown in each of part *A, B, C* and *D.*

- Assessing the activation of the right and left atrium found the following activation sequences:
  - Posterior left atrium—high to low
  - Anterior left atrium—high to low
  - Perimitral activation—septal to lateral anteriorly and posteriorly
  - Right atrium—septal to lateral right atrium
  On the basis of this a macro reentrant tachycardia could be excluded.

Localization of the source of focal-source AT with ATCL 220 milliseconds was then undertaken.

Although more than 2 catheters are not required to diagnose localized reentry, a multipolar mapping catheter can very nicely illustrate the principle behind this form of arrhythmia. **Fig. 6** shows a multielectrode circular mapping catheter in the left atrium demonstrating local activity spanning the entire AT cycle length.

The intracardiac recordings illustrate mapping of the entire AT cycle length (>70%) on the 10 bipoles of the circular mapping catheter covering a surface area of approximately 3 cm², very nicely showing a localized reentry circuit. The activation of the remainder of the atrial chamber occurs from the centrifugal spread of the impulse rotating in this small area.

After activation mapping, the localized reentrant mechanism should be confirmed by entrainment maneuvers.

As shown in **Fig. 7**, the ablation catheter is now at the site where the LASSO had localized the reentry circuit. Because there is now only a single

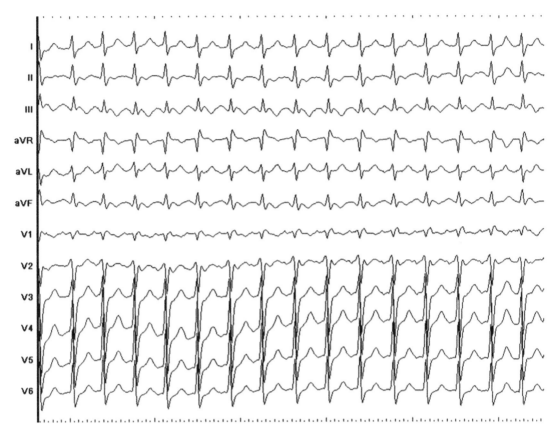

Fig. 5. 12-lead electrocardiogram of an atrial tachycardia with a cycle length of 220 milliseconds and a cycle length variation of less than 5%.

bipole, the recording of the fractionated electrogram now spans 40% to 45% of the ATCL at this single site. Naturally the catheter can be moved gently to map all of the local reentry cycle length.

In **Fig. 8**, the diagnosis is confirmed showing a PPI, after successful entrainment of the tachycardia (<30 milliseconds), suggestive of entrainment location close to the source of AT.

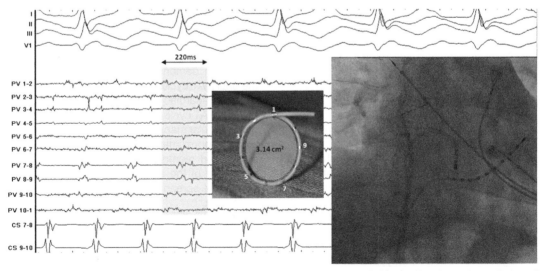

Fig. 6. Multielectrode mapping of a focal-source atrial tachycardia; most of the atrial tachycardia cycle length (>70%) can be seen on the 10 bipoles of the circular catheter.

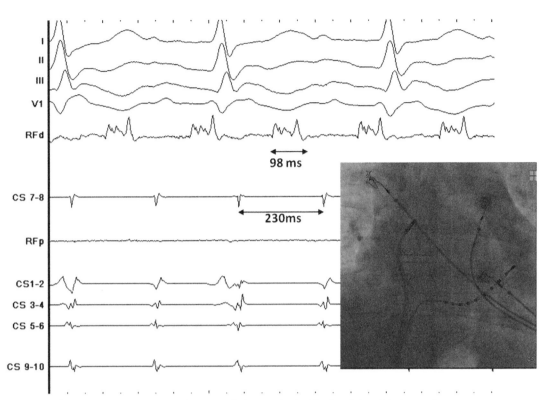

Fig. 7. Localized reentry site potential as recorded on a single bipole of the ablation catheter.

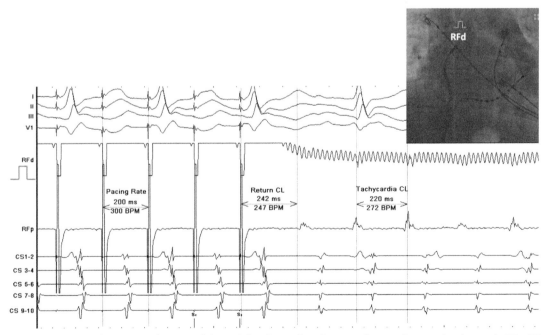

Fig. 8. Confirming the source of origin of the atrial tachycardia using entrainment (postpacing interval <30 milliseconds). CL, cycle length.

SUMMARY

Focal-source ATs are common following AF ablation. They can be hard to map, but with due patience and perseverance, the source of earliest activation can usually be located. It is very useful to first rule out a macro reentrant tachycardia, and following this start, homing in on the source. Once entrainment has confirmed the source of the AT, the target can be ablated.

REFERENCES

1. Jais P, Matsuo S, Knecht S, et al. A deductive mapping strategy for atrial tachycardia following atrial fibrillation ablation: importance of localized reentry. J Cardiovasc Electrophysiol 2009;20(5):480–91.

2. Haissaguerre M, Hocini M, Sanders P, et al. Catheter ablation of long-lasting persistent atrial fibrillation: clinical outcome and mechanisms of subsequent arrhythmias. J Cardiovasc Electrophysiol 2005; 16(11):1138–47.

3. Chae S, Oral H, Good E, et al. Atrial tachycardia after circumferential pulmonary vein ablation of atrial fibrillation. J Am Coll Cardiol 2007;50(18):1781–7.

4. Rostock T, Drewitz I, Steven D, et al. Characterization, mapping, and catheter ablation of recurrent atrial tachycardias after stepwise ablation of long-lasting persistent atrial fibrillation. Circ Arrhythm Electrophysiol 2010;3(2):160–9.

5. Mohamed U, Skanes AC, Gula LJ, et al. A novel pacing maneuver to localize focal atrial tachycardia. J Cardiovasc Electrophysiol 2007;18: 1–6.

Typical Examples of Focal-Source Atrial Tachycardia

Michala Pedersen, MD*, Amir S. Jadidi, MD,
Frederic Sacher, MD, Meleze Hocini, MD

KEYWORDS

• Atrial tachycardia • Focal source • Local reentry • Mapping • Activation • Entrainment

KEY POINTS

- Mapping atrial tachycardias (ATs) depends on understanding the AT electrical propagation (activation mapping) and on entrainment/postpacing intervals (PPI).
- In the case of focal-source ATs, the global electrical mapping and postpacing intervals allow the operator to rule out the macroreentrant ATs and determine that the arrhythmia is compatible with a "centrifugal" AT.
- It can take time and perseverance to map and locate the very earliest potentials.
- An added difficulty often encountered after ablation for atrial fibrillation is that in the region of interest the AT potentials may be masked by freshly ablated tissue (probably because of edema) and, despite very high gains, are difficult to interpret.
- Edema may also explain why it can be difficult to capture for entrainment and why sometimes longer radiofrequency delivery is needed to terminate the arrhythmia.

INTRODUCTION

In this article examples of the mapping of focal source atrial tachycardias (ATs) are presented. The aim is to underpin the strategies for mapping these ATs as described in the other articles in this issue. Each case contains many individual examples of maneuvers. It is worthwhile spending time on each figure and understanding the mapping technique used.

CASE 1

Fig. 1 shows the 12-lead electrocardiogram of an AT with a cycle length (CL) of 218 ms and an AT CL variation of less than 3%. It can also be seen that there is variable block to the ventricle.

Fig. 2 shows the intracardiac signals during the AT, with the ablation catheter near the mitral isthmus on the left and at the septum on the right.

- On activation mapping, the septal and left lateral atrial sites are activated simultaneously. The activation of CS also occurs during the same temporal window.
- The perimitral and the right-sided ATs are ruled out based on such an activation pattern.
- The activation proceeded from high to low on both anterior and posterior walls of the left atrium (LA) (not shown), ruling out a roof-dependent macroreentry AT.

Fig. 3 shows entrainment mapping of the AT. Entrainment mapping can be performed if the AT is very stable; however, many ATs are unstable and indeed terminate or change with entrainment, and as such, activation mapping is usually the safest first strategy.

- On entrainment of the tachycardia from various sites in the left atrium, there was a shorter

---

Conflicts of Interest: None.
Disclosures: None.
Department of Electrophysiology, Hôpital Cardiologique du Haut-Lévêque and the Université Victor Segalen Bordeaux II, Bordeaux, Pessac 33604, France
* Corresponding author. Hôpital Haut Lévêque, Bordeaux, Pessac 33604, France.
E-mail address: michalapedersen@doctors.org.uk

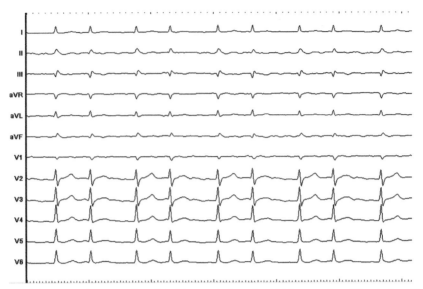

Fig. 1. Twelve-lead electrocardiogram of an AT with a cycle length of 218 ms and an AT cycle length variation of less than 3%.

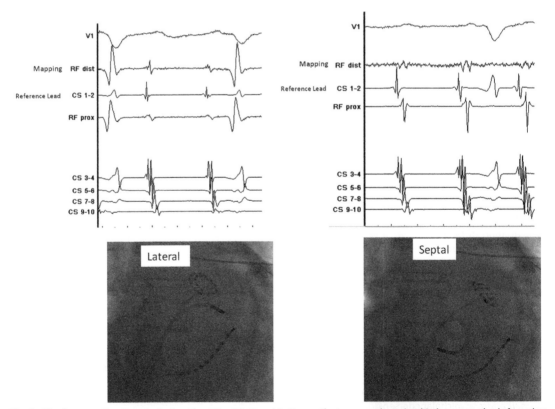

Fig. 2. The intracardiac signals during the AT, with the ablation catheter near the mitral isthmus on the left and at the septum on the right.

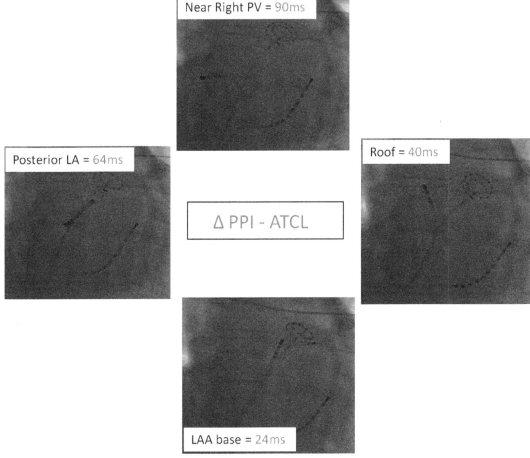

Fig. 3. Entrainment mapping from 4 different sites in the LA, the Δ postpacing interval–AT cycle length (ΔPPI − AT CL) being shortest by the base of the left atrial appendage. LAA, left atrial appendage; PV, pulmonary veins.

ΔPPI − AT CL interval moving toward the left atrial appendage from the right pulmonary veins.

- This was suggestive of focal-source AT near the superior left pulmonary vein–left atrial appendage area.

In **Fig. 4**, the spiral catheter was moved to the superior left pulmonary vein–left atrial appendage area and was gently moved around to try map the source of the AT.

- Almost the entire AT cycle length was recorded on the bipoles of the spiral catheter (as highlighted in the figure). This spiral catheter was noted at the junction of the left appendage and roof area.
- Localized reentry was successfully diagnosed and ablated in this region.
- In usual circumstances, high-density mapping catheters, like the spiral catheter, are not used during AT, but they can prove very helpful indeed.
- Ablation in this area terminated the tachycardia

CASE 2

During a long ablation case of persistent atrial fibrillation (AF), the AF finally terminated to an AT with a cycle length of 256 ms, as shown in **Fig. 5**.

Fig. 6 illustrates a cycle-length variation from 252 to 260 ms, giving a cycle length variation of 3%.

In **Fig. 7**, the left-hand panel shows distal to proximal activation on the CS catheter. The middle and right-hand panels show that the ablation catheter is at the septum and laterally near the mitral isthmus, respectively.

- Activation mapping reveals lateral to septal activation of both the posterior wall (CS) and the anterior wall of the left atrium.

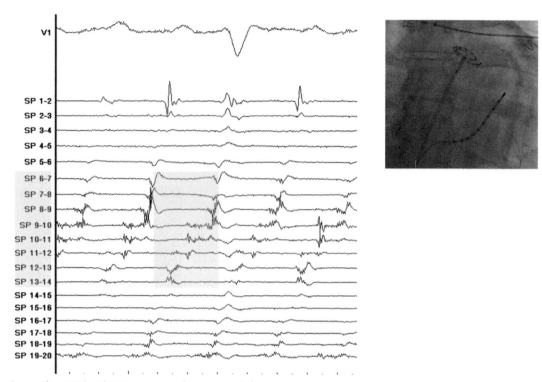

Fig. 4. The spiral catheter is now at the superior left pulmonary vein–left atrial appendage area, aiming to map the source of the AT.

- Perimitral and right ATs are therefore most unlikely at this stage.

Figs. 8 and **9** show the ablation catheter mapping the direction of activation between high and low on the on the posterior and anterior walls.

- Activation mapping of the anterior and posterior LA walls occur at the same time

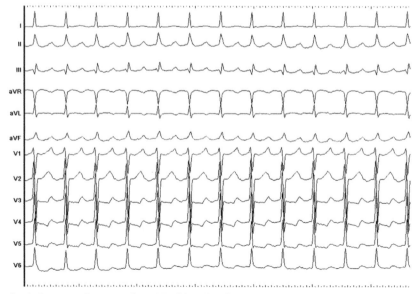

Fig. 5. Twelve-lead electrocardiogram of an AT with a CL of 256 ms.

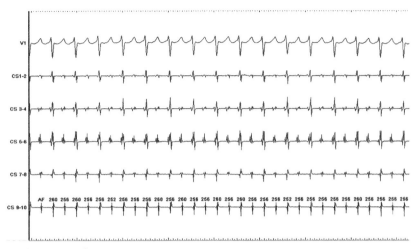

Fig. 6. Cycle length variation from 252 ms to 260 ms.

and in the same directions (from low to high).

- Such an activation pattern is not compatible with roof-dependent reentry.

In **Fig. 10**, entrainment from the lateral right atrium is displayed.

In **Fig. 11**, entrainment from the lateral left atrium is shown.

Fig. 12 displays entrainment from the posterior left atrium.

- Entrainment mapping from lateral right and lateral left atria revealed long ΔPPI − AT CL. The shortest ΔPPI − AT CL was obtained on the low posterior left atrium.
- Based on the findings of entrainment mapping, the focal source of the AT was diagnosed to be within the low posterior left atrial segment.

Fig. 13 shows a multi-electrode catheter at the low posterior left atrial segment.

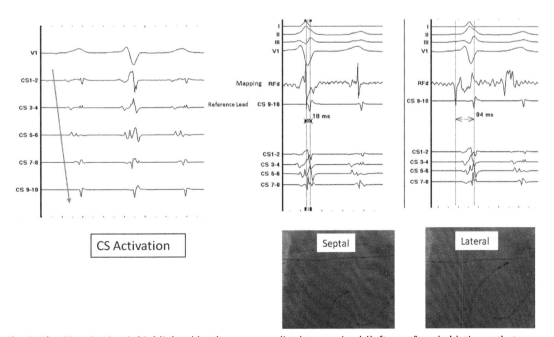

Fig. 7. The CS activation is highlighted by the arrow as distal to proximal (*left panel*) and ablation catheter are placed at the septum and laterally near the mitral isthmus (*middle* and *right panels*, respectively).

220

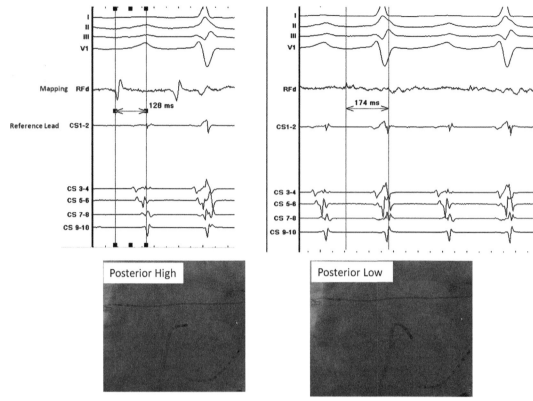

Fig. 8. Activation mapping of the posterior wall.

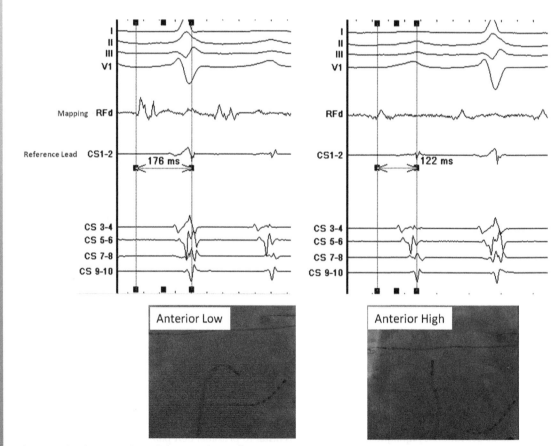

Fig. 9. Activation mapping of the anterior wall.

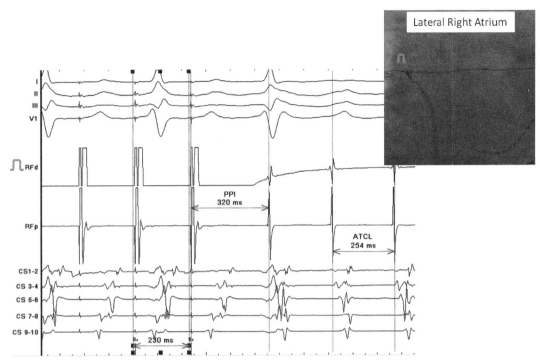

Fig. 10. Entrainment from the lateral right atrium.

- Due to the extensive defragmentation ablation, the amplitude of the electrograms of the posterior wall was too low to achieve clear mapping or to prove arrhythmia localization and mechanism. A multi-electrode catheter (at scale of ×32) was therefore added to aid mapping the posterior wall and these localized small consistent potentials at the posterior wall.
- Mapping around the lasso with the ablation catheter could not provide any earlier activation, confirming the origin of the centrifugal tachycardia in the posterior wall.

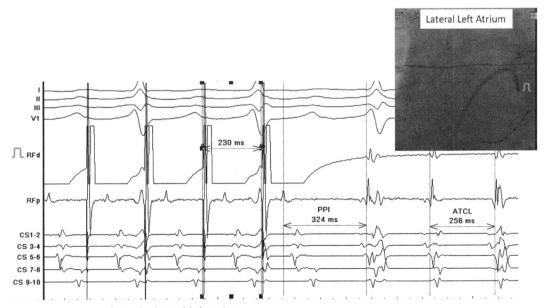

Fig. 11. Entrainment from the lateral left atrium.

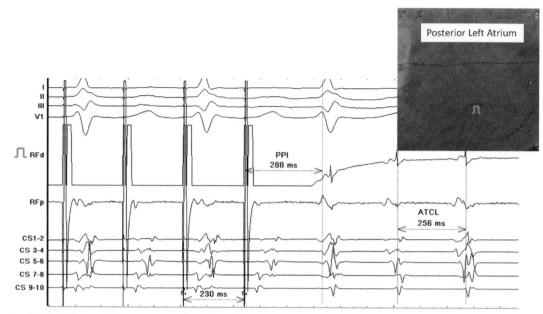

Fig. 12. Entrainment from the posterior left atrium.

Fig. 14 shows the ablation catheter at the area of interest.

- Consistent potentials suggestive of an AT were barely present. The authors ablated this area mainly guided by their knowledge of the global electrical mapping of the LA activation. Despite the absence of significant potentials at the ablation site, the AT

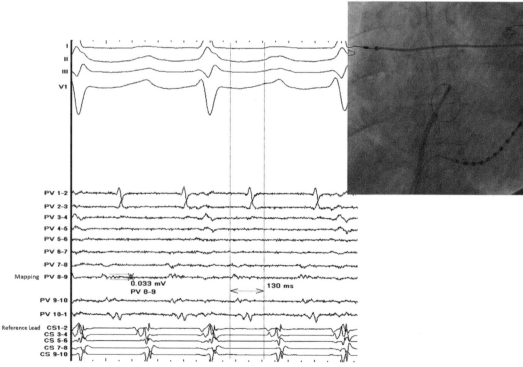

Fig. 13. A multi-electrode catheter at the low posterior left atrial segment to help mapping the area of interest.

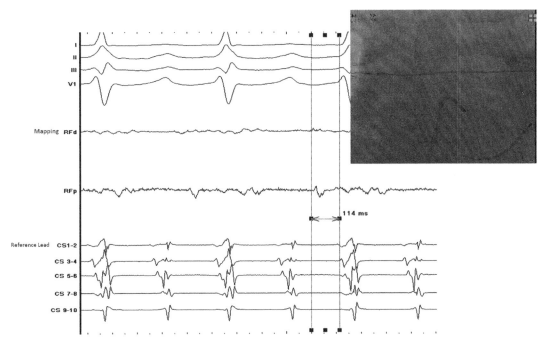

Fig. 14. The ablation catheter at the area of interest.

terminated within 53 seconds of ablation and was subsequently noninducible.

Fig. 15; Termination of the tachycardia with radiofrequency (RF) delivery.

- In this case, the global electrical mapping and postpacing intervals allowed us to determine that the arrhythmia was compatible with a focal-source AT, centrifugally spreading to the rest of the atrium.

- In the region of interest, the AT potentials were masked in the freshly ablated tissue (probably because of edema) and, despite very high gains, difficult to interpret. Edema may also explain why the AT needed a full 53 seconds of RF to terminate.
- This case highlights the difficulty in mapping (and ablating) the left atrium following extensive RF delivery, such as after ablation for persistent AF.

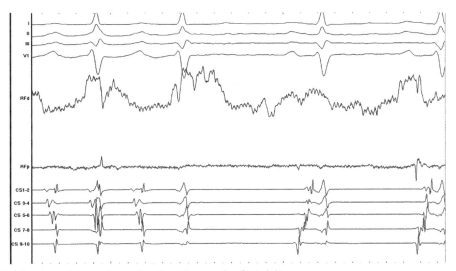

Fig. 15. Termination of the tachycardia after 53 seconds of RF delivery.

SUMMARY

Mapping ATs depends on understanding the AT electrical propagation (activation mapping) and on entrainment/postpacing intervals. In the case of focal-source ATs, the global electrical mapping and postpacing intervals allow the operator to rule out the macroreentrant ATs and determine that the arrhythmia is compatible with a "centrifugal" AT. The next step is to localize the region of interest and then pinpoint the earliest potentials.

It can take time and perseverance to map and locate the very earliest potentials. The last example shows an added difficulty often encountered after ablation for atrial fibrillation; in the region of interest, the AT potentials may be masked by freshly ablated tissue (probably because of edema) and, despite very high gains, difficult to interpret. Edema may also explain why it can be difficult to capture for entrainment and why sometimes longer RF delivery is needed to terminate the arrhythmia.

Misleading Features of Activation and Entrainment Mapping

Ashok J. Shah, MD[a,b],*, Shinsuke Miyazaki, MD[a,b],
Xing-Peng Liu, MD[a,b], Yuki Komatsu, MD[a,b],
Patrizio Pascale, MD[a,b], Pierre Jais, MD[a,b]

KEYWORDS

• Atrial tachycardia • Activation • Entrainment • Atypical feature

KEY POINTS

- Recognition of endocardial left atrial (LA) activation occurring in a different direction from the more obvious local coronary sinus (CS) activation is critical to avoid misleading interpretations during mapping of atrial tachycardia (AT).
- Short return cycle during entrainment mapping maneuver may or may not be true return cycle. If it is not a real return cycle (but the last captured beat), it may be due to far-field capture phenomenon or delayed local capture.
- Far-field capture phenomenon can be differentiated from delayed local capture by recognizing that the pacing site is the last activated bipole. On the contrary, the pacing site is the first activated site in delayed local capture.
- In far-field capture phenomenon, pacing site is activated the last because the high/maximum output pacing stimulus gets delivered during its refractory period and results in capture of the excitable gap that has just passed past it.
- A long return cycle (postpacing interval [PPI]) after entrainment from a site lying close to the macro-reentry circuit can be encountered because of altered local conduction properties.

INTRODUCTION

Activation and entrainment maneuvers constitute the basic tools of a diagnostic mapping process using a combination of the following catheters during an electrophysiological procedure for ablation of ATs after atrial fibrillation (AF) ablation:

1. A deflectable decapolar catheter (5-mm interelectrode spacing, Xtrem, Sorin, France) positioned within the CS with the distal electrode positioned at 4 o'clock position along the mitral annulus in the 30° left anterior oblique radiographic projection.

2. A 3.5 mm externally irrigated-tip quadripolar ablation catheter (5-mm interelectrode spacing, Thermocool, Biosense Webster Inc, CA, USA).

A decapolar catheter positioned in the CS and a 3.5-mm-tip quadripolar ablation catheter introduced through the long sheath would suffice for mapping and ablation of most ATs.

This article describes the following atypical features of activation and entrainment encountered during the diagnostic mapping of ATs:

- CS activation is a good surrogate for the contiguous endocardial LA activation in

Conflicts of Interest: None.
Disclosures: None.
[a] Department of Rhythmologie, Hôpital Cardiologique du Haut-Lévêque; [b] Department of Rhythmologie, Université Victor Segalen Bordeaux II, Bordeaux, France
* Corresponding author. Department of Rhythmologie, Hôpital Haut Lévêque, 33604 Bordeaux-Pessac, France.
E-mail address: drashahep@gmail.com

most situations. Atypically, CS activation may not represent the activation of the contiguous LA. In such situations, one needs to carefully evaluate the CS electrograms and distinguish them from those of the LA to decipher the activation of the regional LA.

- Not very unusually after successful entrainment of AT, the return cycle (PPI) is found to be shorter than the tachycardia cycle length (TCL). Such an atypical characteristic of entrainment mapping may be due to delayed local capture or far-field capture phenomenon.
- A long return cycle (PPI) after entrainment from a site lying close to the macroreentry circuit can be encountered because of altered local conduction.

ATYPICAL CS ACTIVATION PATTERN

Disparity in the activation of CS and contiguous LA is illustrated in a patient with post-AF ablation AT at 530 ms cycle length.[1] The 12-lead ECG shown in **Fig. 1** displays an isoelectric line between the 2 successive P waves during tachycardia, which indicates the mechanism of this AT as either a focal activity or a macroreentry with very slowly conducting isthmus that could have emerged from multiple previous ablations.

As shown in **Fig. 2**, CS activation occurred in the distal to proximal direction, that is, from CS 1-2 to CS 5-6, and also in the proximal to distal direction, that is, from CS 9-10 to CS 7-8. On further activation mapping (not shown), it was observed that the activation of the anterior and the posterior LA walls occurred from below upward (low to high). On entrainment mapping of the tachycardia, it could be entrained successfully from the anterolateral and anteroseptal LA. The PPI from each of these sites equaled the TCL (530 ms) (**Fig. 3**). The low to high pattern of activation of the anterior and posterior walls and Δ PPI − TCL = 0 from 2 opposite sides of the mitral annulus established the diagnosis of macroreentry around the mitral annulus. Mitral isthmus linear ablation resulted in termination of tachycardia and successful restoration of sinus rhythm, thereby confirming the diagnosis of perimitral flutter. However, the CS activation pattern did not fit with the diagnosis of perimitral flutter, considering CS as an inevitable anatomic part of the perimitral reentrant circuit. On normal scale, CS activation was inconsistent with perimitral macroreentry. At twice the magnification of the normal scale on all the CS bipoles during tachycardia (**Fig. 4**), tiny far-field potentials, which originated from the LA, were identified distinctly from the near-field CS electrograms. These potentials represented the counterclockwise tachycardia-related concentric activation of the LA area contiguous to the CS. CS bipoles 1-2 to 5-6 were bystanders during perimitral flutter and therefore, their activation, which was in the opposite direction to that of the far-field LA activity, did not concur with perimitral activation pattern. Contiguous LA was forming the posterior half of perimitral circuit in this patient. Far-field LA potentials may not visualized clearly on the CS bipoles at the usual magnification scale (**Box 1**).

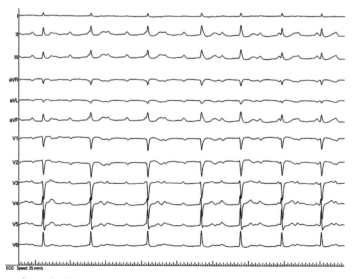

Fig. 1. A 12-Lead ECG of atrial tachycardia.

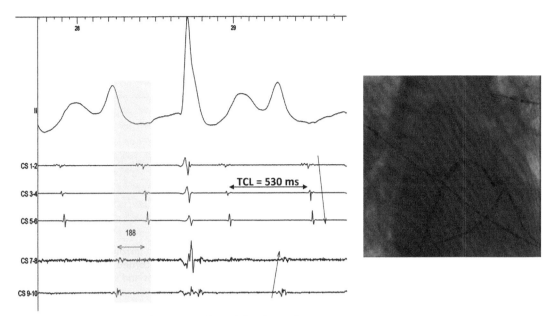

Fig. 2. Coronary sinus activation pattern in atrial tachycardia.

Pascale and colleagues[3] studied 149 ATs post-AF ablation. Disparate LA-CS activations were apparent in 20 (13%) ATs after magnifying the CS recording scale. The most common (90%) pattern was distal to proximal endocardial LA activation against proximal to distal CS activation, the latter involving the whole CS or its distal part. Perimitral macroreentry was more common when disparate LA-CS activation was observed than when it was not observed (67% vs 29%; $P = .002$).

In another example of perimitral AT at 230 ms, shown in **Fig. 5**, distal CS activation occurs with every alternate tachycardia beat, suggesting 2:1 conduction of AT into the distal CS. Far-field LA potentials recorded on the CS catheter occur in 1:1 relationship with the tachycardia, suggesting passive activation of CS during the tachycardia.[4] This example underscores the importance of far-field and therefore relatively smaller LA signals recorded on the epicardially located CS catheter during LA tachycardia. Careful analysis of CS recordings during AT after AF ablation is critical to avoid misleading interpretations of activation maps of AT. On a wider clinical scale, it is

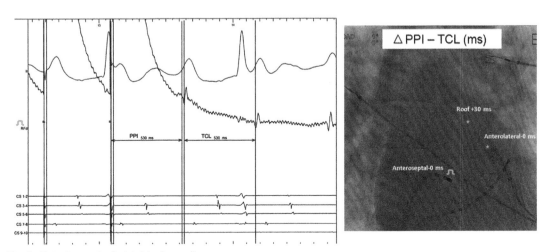

Fig. 3. Entrainment of atrial tachycardia.

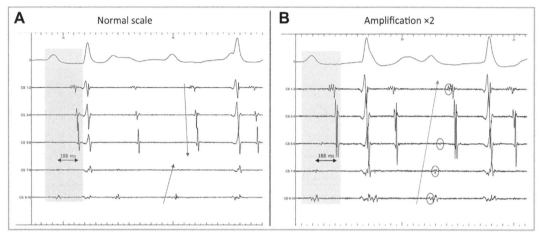

Fig. 4. (*A*) Coronary sinus electrograms at normal scale show the activation pattern (*arrows*) during tachycardia. (*B*) At twice the magnification of the normal scale, the left atrial electrograms recorded on the coronary sinus catheter stand out separately (*encircled*) from the local coronary sinus electrograms and show a distinct pattern of activation (*arrow*) from the coronary sinus.

important to recognize this atypical feature of activation for appropriate assessment of left mitral isthmus block by differential CS and left appendage pacing maneuvers.[5]

ATYPICAL ENTRAINMENT FEATURE: SHORT RETURN CYCLE

After successful entrainment of AT, the PPI is shorter than the TCL if there is delay in local capture or a far-field capture phenomenon happens. The latter is explained in detail below.

For the AT at 255 ms (**Fig. 6**), entrainment of tachycardia from distal bipole of the mapping/ablation catheter (radiofrequency distal [RFd]) at 240 ms results in amplifier saturation (asterisk), disallowing interpretation of PPI from the pacing

---

Box 1
Learning points

- In 2% perimitral AT, CS activation is neither proximal to distal nor distal to proximal.[2]
- Far-field LA potentials should always be looked for, and if they are visible distinctly from the CS potentials, they should be considered as representative of the inferoposterior LA activation. CS may not always be a part of the perimitral circuit.
- Final diagnosis of AT should be based on activation sequence and entrainment maneuvers.

---

bipole (RFd).[6] The proximal bipole (radiofrequency proximal [RFp]) may be considered as a proxy of RFd and is used for the measurement of PPI. The PPI measured on RFp was 184 ms and was shorter than the TCL (255 ms).

As shown in **Fig. 7**, the possibility of delayed local capture can be ruled out because the last entrained beat results in activation of the CS bipoles earlier than that of the RFp, the proxy for the pacing electrode. If there was a delayed local capture, CS bipoles would have been activated later than the pacing electrode.

Fig. 7 also shows that, during entrainment, the stimulus to local electrogram delay on RFp was 184 ms. Thus the electrogram, which follows the last pacing stimulus on the RFp, is not the first returning beat of the tachycardia (commonly called "return cycle") but the last entrained beat. The PPI, which is measured from the last entrained beat to the first return AT cycle, is 255 ms and is equal to the TCL. Thus, the pacing site (Radiofrequency [RF]) is lying within the tachycardia circuit. Now for the answer to the intriguing question, why is the pacing electrode the last activated site during tachycardia entrainment undertaken from the site within the tachycardia circuit.

The concept of far-field capture is explained using the diagrams in **Figs. 8–11**. **Fig. 8** shows that the size of the virtual electrode varies with the strength of the pacing output during entrainment pacing from a site within or close to the reentrant tachycardia circuit. In this situation, when the maximum-output pacing is undertaken, the following features ensue (see **Fig. 9**).

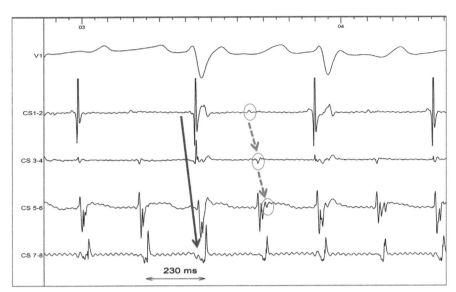

Fig. 5. Importance of left atrial activation recorded on the coronary sinus catheter.

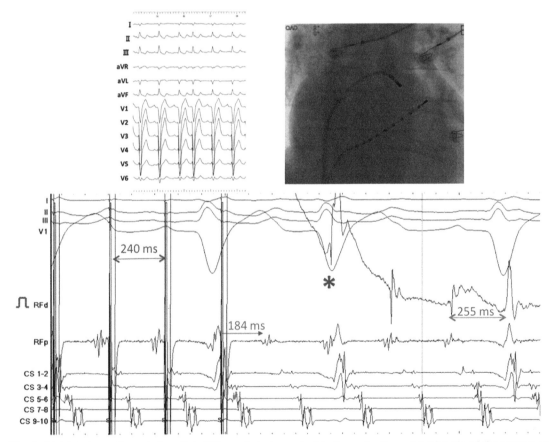

Fig. 6. Atrial tachycardia cycle length is 255 ms. Entrainment of tachycardia from distal bipole of the mapping/ablation catheter (RFd) at 240 ms results in amplifier saturation (*asterisk*) disallowing interpretation of post pacing interval from the pacing bipole (RFd). The postpacing interval measured on the proxy electrode (RFp) seems to be 184 ms. It is shorter than the tachycardia cycle length (255 ms). On careful observation, this postpacing interval is actually representing the last captured beat. Abbreviations: RFd, radiofrequency distal; RFp, radiofrequency proximal.

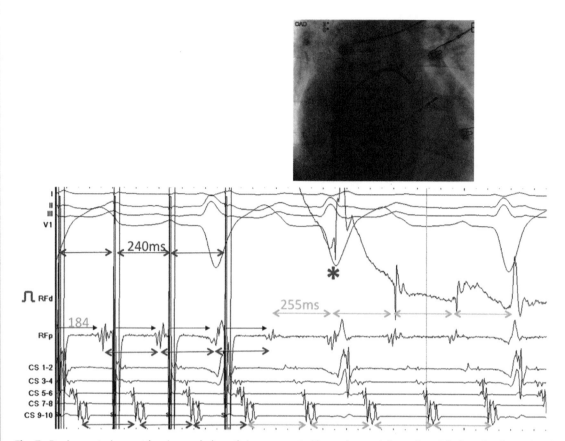

Fig. 7. During entrainment (pacing cycle length is represented by *red arrow*) from the RFd, the stimulus to local electrogram delay (*blue arrow*) on RFp is 184 ms. The last entrained beat results in activation of the coronary sinus bipoles earlier than that of the RFp, the proxy for the pacing electrode. This rules out delayed local capture. The electrogram, which follows the last pacing stimulus on the RFp is not the first returning beat of the tachycardia but the last entrained beat. The post-pacing interval on RFp is 255 ms and equal to the tachycardia cycle length (*green arrow*). Asterisk represents the first visible electrical activity on RFd post pacing.

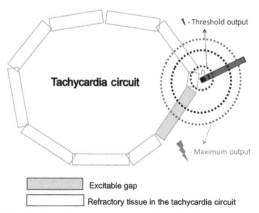

Fig. 8. Entrainment pacing: virtual electrode size varies with pacing output.

1. When local tissue is refractory, any strength of pacing output (including the maximum output) does not yield local capture. Thus, the situation in which there is an absence of local capture is generated.

2. However, instead of a local tissue, a wide area of surrounding tissue in the excitable gap is simultaneously captured, which constitutes "far-field capture without local capture."

3. A part of excitable gap remains at the edge of the virtual electrode and allows propagation of wave front along the tachycardia circuit during entrainment pacing.

Furthermore, in **Figs. 10** and **11**,

4. There is a temporal difference in the propagation of activation during "local capture"

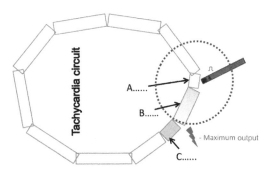

Fig. 9. Concept of far-field capture without local capture.

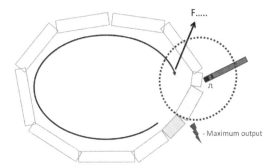

Fig. 11. Passive/last activation at pacing site: evidence of entrainment without local capture.

(whenever it occurs) from that during "far-field capture without local capture."

5. Local activation on the remote recording bipoles is advanced during far-field capture when compared with the local capture.
6. Local activation of the initially refractory pacing site occurs last, that is, after the time it takes for the propagating orthodromic wave front to travel over the tachycardia circuit. Also, far-field capture without local capture will advance the passively activated pacing site.

In summary, if the site lying within the tachycardia circuit is pace-stimulated shortly after it is activated by the tachycardia impulse, it will be refractory to the pacing stimulus. If the pacing stimulus with highest output (maximum strength and therefore widest virtual electrode size) is applied, it could result in capture of the excitable gap, which would have just passed beyond the pacing site. If the entrainment ensues, the local activation will be advanced all along the circuit. Also, the pacing site will be the last activated site instead of the first. **Fig. 12** shows a clinical example (also refer to

Fig. 6) of maximum-output pacing during local refractoriness, which results in far-field capture without local capture. The onset of entrainment maneuver is shown in **Fig. 12**. The first pacing beat (filled yellow arrow) falls in the refractory period of the RFd (see RFp) but still results in the entrainment of the AT as evidenced by advancement of the CS electrograms and that at RFp. Also, as shown in **Fig. 7**, the pacing electrode is the last activated site (because it was not immediately captured) during entrainment, which is explained by the far-field capture phenomenon described above.

Differences Between Far-field Capture Phenomenon and Delayed Local Capture

An example of an apparently similar phenomenon—"delayed local capture"—is shown in **Fig. 13** to highlight its differences from far-field capture phenomenon. AT at 200 ms (cycle length) is entrained at pacing rate of 175 ms. The pacing site is activated (captured) after delay (56 ms) from the stimulus. However, it is still the first activated site during the entrainment of AT. The activation of remote recording sites (electrograms recorded on the CS catheter) follows that of the pacing site. This is completely reversed during far-field capture phenomenon wherein the pacing site is the last activated site.

In **Figs. 14** and **15**, another clinical example of far-field capture, an atypical feature of entrainment mapping characterized by short return cycle, is described.

Far-field capture phenomenon occurs during AT at 290 ms entrained at 260 ms. Amplifier saturation is observed on the pacing bipole: RFd. Shorter return cycle length is observed on the proxy electrode: RFp. The stimulus to local electrogram on RFp is 240 ms, which helps to diagnose the first return cycle electrogram on RFp as the last captured

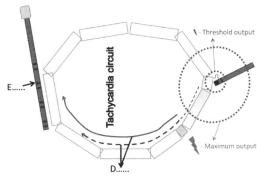

Fig. 10. Advancement of local activation: evidence of entrainment with far-field capture.

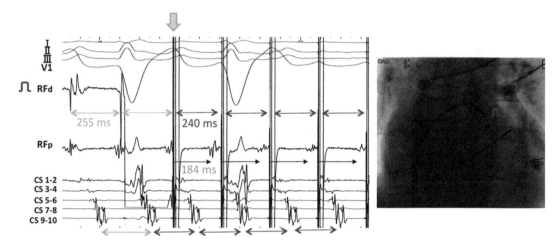

Fig. 12. The onset of entrainment maneuver, which has been shown in **Figs. 6** and **7**. The first pacing beat (*filled yellow arrow*) falls in the refractory period of the RFd (see RFp) but still results in the entrainment of the AT as evidenced by advancement of the CS electrograms and that at RFp. The RFp activation occurs 184 ms after the stimulus.

beat. The actual PPI is equal to TCL when measured from the last captured beat on RFp. The pacing bipole (RFp) is the last activated bipole. The CS bipoles can be seen getting activated earlier than the pacing bipole.

In **Fig. 15**, the onset of entrainment at 260 ms is shown during AT at 290 ms. Amplifier saturation is observed on the pacing bipole: RFd. RFp is regarded as the proxy electrode. The first 4 beats (counted rightward from filled yellow arrow) fall in

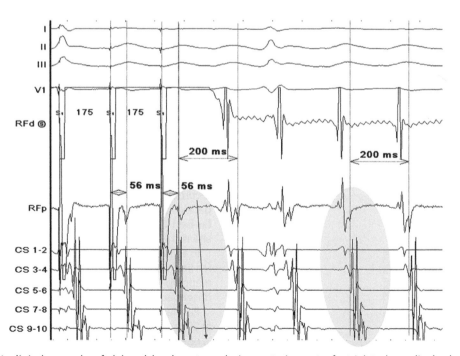

Fig. 13. A clinical example of delayed local capture during entrainment of atrial tachycardia (cycle length 200 ms). The pacing cycle length is 175 ms. The pacing site (RFd/RFp) is activated (captured) after delay (56 ms) from the stimulus. However, it is still the first activated site and precedes the activation of the coronary sinus.

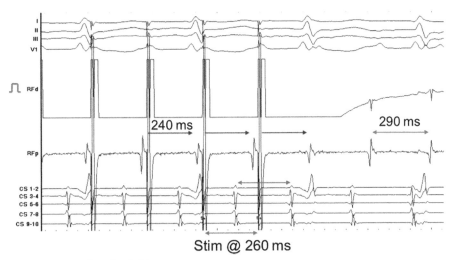

Fig. 14. Entrainment mapping: far-field capture.

the refractory period of the RFp electrical signal, disallowing AT entrainment. Fifth pacing beat (star) falls 40 ms after the local signal on RFp. The excitable gap would have just passed past the RFp allowing capture of the tissue in the excitable gap as evidenced by the advancement of the next RFp signal (270 ms). All CS bipoles are advanced before the RFp. Thus RFp signal happens to be the latest activation site despite itself being the pacing site (proxy). Because it was refractory when the pacing stimulus was applied, it was not

captured and got activated passively, which proves that pacing resulted in capture of the relatively farther tissue while the local pacing site was refractory. This is diagnostic of far-field capture phenomenon (**Box 2**).

ATYPICAL ENTRAINMENT FEATURE: LONG RETURN CYCLE

A long return cycle (PPI) after entrainment from a site lying close to the macroreentry circuit can

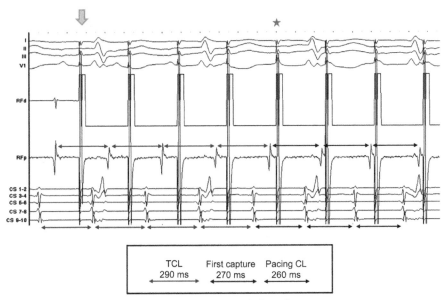

TCL	First capture	Pacing CL
290 ms	270 ms	260 ms

Fig. 15. Entrainment mapping: onset of entrainment. CL, cycle length.

be encountered because of altered local conduction properties. In the 3D electroanatomic map shown in **Fig. 16**, the tachycardia activation pattern is consistent with roof-dependent AT. Entrainment from 2 sites on the anterior LA roof yielded PPIs longer than the TCL by 5 ms and 45 ms, respectively. Entrainment from another segment of macroreentrant circuit was undertaken to confirm the diagnosis of roof-dependent macroreentry (not shown). Having confirmed macroreentry through the roof and because both the spots lie on the roof (close to the reentrant circuit), the expected difference between the PPI and ATCL (Atrial tachycardia cycle length) was 30 ms or less at both the spots. Even when both spots lie in physical proximity to the circuit running through the roof, only one of the 2 spots could be considered lying close to it while strictly applying the criterion of PPI − ATCL ≤30 ms. The reason for longer return cycle at the other pacing site on the roof is slower conduction velocity in the region between the circuit and the pacing site. Despite not being physically far from the roof-dependent circuit, the impulse travels slowly between the pacing spot and the AT circuit taking at least 15 ms longer to traverse the slow zone in recto-verso directions than the usual maximum of 30 ms.

This clinical illustration shows the importance of entrainment from 2 or more distinct/distant segments and the need for its careful interpretation to avoid conflicting the diagnosis of macroreentry with localized reentry.

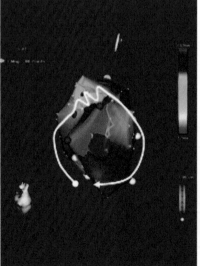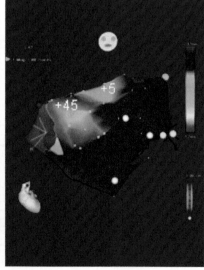

Fig. 16. A 3D electroanatomic map of AT showing activation pattern consistent with roof-dependent tachycardia. The entrainment mapping from 2 sites on the anterior roof yielded postpacing interval longer than tachycardia cycle length by 5 ms and 45 ms, respectively.

SUMMARY

Atypical activation and entrainment characteristics can lead to inappropriate interpretation of these critical maneuvers, which may cause diagnostic difficulties during tachycardia mapping. The timely recognition of these important clinically encountered features is feasible with due diligence.

REFERENCES

1. Shah AJ, Jadidi AS, Liu X, et al. Eccentric activation of coronary sinus during perimitral flutter is a rare phenomenon: what is the mechanism? J Cardiovasc Electrophysiol 2011;22(3):354–8.
2. Jais P, Matsuo S, Knecht S, et al. A deductive mapping strategy for atrial tachycardia following atrial fibrillation ablation: importance of localized reentry. J Cardiovasc Electrophysiol 2009;20(5): 480–91.
3. Pascale P, Shah AJ, Roten L, et al. Disparate activation of the coronary sinus and inferior left atrium during atrial tachycardia after persistent atrial fibrillation ablation: prevalence, pitfalls, and impact on mapping. J Cardiovasc Electrophysiol 2012;23(7): 697–707.
4. Jadidi AS, Shah AJ, Miyazaki S, et al. Changing activation pattern of the coronary sinus during ongoing perimitral flutter. J Cardiovasc Electrophysiol 2012; 23(4):445–6.
5. Shah AJ, Pascale P, Miyazaki S, et al. Prevalence and types of pitfall in the assessment of mitral isthmus linear conduction block. Circ Arrhythm Electrophysiol 2012;5(5):957–67.
6. Miyazaki S, Shah A, Liu X, et al. Entrainment mapping of perimitral flutter. J Cardiovasc Electrophysiol 2011; 22(1):101–3.

Exotic Atrial Tachycardias

Ashok J. Shah, MD*, Shinsuke Miyazaki, MD,
Sebastien Knecht, MD, Seiichiro Matsuo, MD,
Matthew Daly, MD, Yuki Komatsu, MD,
Patrizio Pascale, MD, Laurent Roten, MD,
Meleze Hocini, MD

KEYWORDS

• Dual atrial tachycardia • Double loop • Incarcerated focal source • Localized reentry • Exotic

KEY POINTS

- Catheter ablation of atrial fibrillation can tightly compartmentalize biatrial chamber like a surgical ablation procedure.
- Clinical coexistence of 2 organized atrial rhythms (sinus rhythm and tachycardia or 2 tachycardias with the same or different mechanisms) is rare but not impossible after an ablation procedure.
- Despite restoration of sinus rhythm globally, the tachycardia may not be eliminated and can persist in the incarcerated focal source.
- Activation mapping can suggest a diagnosis of macroreentry but cannot differentiate it from localized reentry arising near the blocked linear lesion.
- Entrainment mapping maneuver is necessary to confirm macroreentry suggested by activation mapping.

INTRODUCTION

Atrial tachycardias (ATs) arising in the context of catheter ablation of atrial fibrillation (AF) require a systematic approach for successful ablation and long-lasting remission. In an electrophysiologic laboratory, these arrhythmias display unique characteristics. They are frequently more than 1 in number, such that progress toward sinus rhythm encompasses multiple forms of AT.[1] They can manifest in rapid succession as ablation converts subtly 1 form to another. They can be very fast to very slow. Because they are often recurrent or incessant and drug resistant and leave patients with more unbearable symptoms than AF, ablation is considered the first-line therapy. Besides a systematic diagnostic approach, these arrhythmias require ablation at the appropriate sites because random ablation can be proarrhythmic and can also hamper the appropriate diagnosis.

This article discuses some unusual forms of clinical ATs encountered after AF ablation:

1. Dual ATs (simultaneous focal and macroreentrant ATs)
2. Double-loop AT (2 simultaneous macroreentrant ATs)
3. Incarcerated focal AT
4. Localized reentrant AT mimicking macroreentry (focal AT arising from near the blocked linear lesion)

DUAL AT (SIMULTANEOUS AND INDEPENDENT FOCAL AND MACROREENTRANT ATS)

Fig. 1 shows a 12-lead electrocardiogram (ECG) undertaken at the start of an AT mapping and ablation procedure, showing clinical AT at 200 milliseconds with less than 10% variation in cycle length.[2]

Conflicts of interest: None.
Disclosures: None.
Hôpital Cardiologique du Haut-Lévêque and the Université Victor Segalen Bordeaux II, Bordeaux, France
* Corresponding author. Department of Rhythmologie and Service of Pr Haissaguerre, Hôpital Cardiologique du Haut Lévêque, Avenue de Magellan, Pessac-Bordeaux 33604, France.
E-mail address: drashahep@gmail.com

Card Electrophysiol Clin 5 (2013) 237–251
http://dx.doi.org/10.1016/j.ccep.2013.02.001
1877-9182/13/$ – see front matter © 2013 Elsevier Inc. All rights reserved.

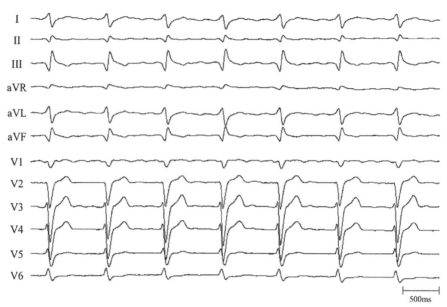

Fig. 1. AT, 12-lead electrocardiogram (ECG). Cycle length, 200 milliseconds; variation, 10%.

Fig. 2 shows intracardiac recordings during an electrophysiologic study using 2 catheters. The activation of all the bipoles except bipole 1-2 of a decapolar CS catheter occurs at 200 milliseconds. CS 1-2 is consistently activated at 150 milliseconds, suggesting dissociation from the rest of the CS bipoles. Even during tachycardia entrainment maneuvers from the lateral right atrium shown in **Fig. 3** and the low septal right atrium shown in **Fig. 4**, CS 1-2 remains dissociated. All other bipoles of the CS are entrained.

High-density Mapping

During high-density mapping with a 20-pole multispline catheter in the right inferior pulmonary vein ostium, rapid venous firing from 75 milliseconds

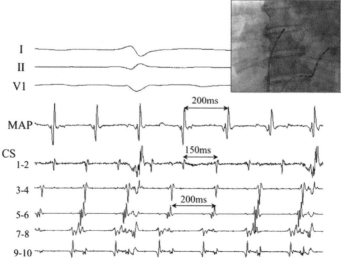

Fig. 2. Activation out of phase on distal CS bipoles.

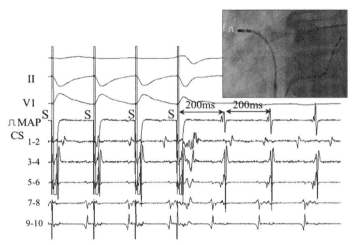

Fig. 3. Entrainment mapping, lateral right atrium.

cycle length (eg, splines A-p and E-p) is recorded as shown in **Fig. 5**. There is 2:1 conduction from the vein to the ostium (eg, splines A-d, B, D, and E-d). CS proximal bipole remains out of phase with the recordings on the multispline catheter but in phase with the far-field right atrial activity (red star) at 200 milliseconds recorded on spline D.

On further mapping in the right atrium, the tachycardia at 200 milliseconds was diagnosed to be peritricuspid macroreentry. Focal pulmonary vein tachycardia at 75 milliseconds was independently driving some portion of the left atrium at

150 milliseconds. Thus, there are 2 independent tachycardias simultaneously driving 2 different atrial chambers at 2 different rates.

Like the surgical maze procedure, catheter ablation of AF can also tightly compartmentalize the biatrial chamber as shown in **Fig. 6** (red circles, red lines, and red dots).

DOUBLE-LOOP AT (2 SIMULTANEOUS MACROREENTRANT ATS)

Fig. 7 shows a 12-lead ECG of clinical AT at 274 milliseconds and cycle length variation less

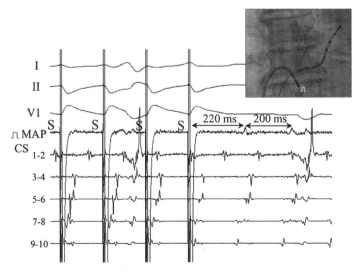

Fig. 4. Entrainment mapping, low septal right atrium.

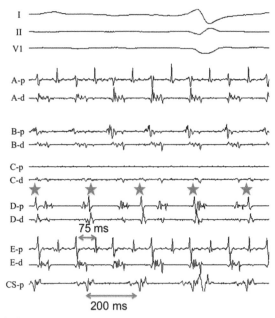
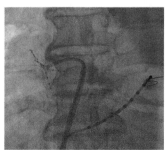

Fig. 5. High-density mapping.

than 5%. Activation mapping around the mitral annulus was consistent with counterclockwise perimitral flutter, as shown in **Fig. 8**.

Entrainment is the confirmatory maneuver when an activation pattern is diagnostic of macroreentry. Tachycardia was entrained from low left septum and distal coronary sinus, which yielded a postpacing interval (PPI) equal to tachycardia cycle length (TCL) at each of the 2 sites, as shown in **Figs. 9** and **10**, respectively. The right panel of

Fig. 10 also shows the outcome of tachycardia entrainment from the right atrium, confirming that the right atrium did not form part of the tachycardia circuit of counterclockwise perimitral flutter.

Fig. 11 shows the tachycardia entrainment results from the anterior and posterior left atrium. The PPI minus TCL was less than 30 milliseconds at both the sites, which indicated that high anterolateral and high posterior left atrial pacing sites also formed a part of the tachycardia circuit.

Activation and entrainment mapping of tachycardia was consistent with perimitral flutter. High lateral and posterior left atrial entrainment mapping revealed that these sites were also lying within or close to the macroreentrant circuit. Hence, the diagnosis was double-loop tachycardia (**Fig. 12**) with 2 coexisting circuits:

1. Around the mitral annulus (perimitral AT)
2. Around the circumferential lesion encircling the pulmonary veins (roof-dependent AT)

Considering that the roof line is easier to draw than the mitral isthmus line, roof ablation was started to terminate the roof-dependent AT, as shown in **Fig. 13**. ATCL prolonged from 274 milliseconds (278 milliseconds in the figure) to 290 milliseconds after 74seconds of linear ablation. Prolongation of ATCL to 290 milliseconds resulted from termination of roof-dependent flutter

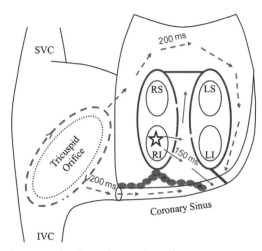

Fig. 6. Dual independent tachycardias.

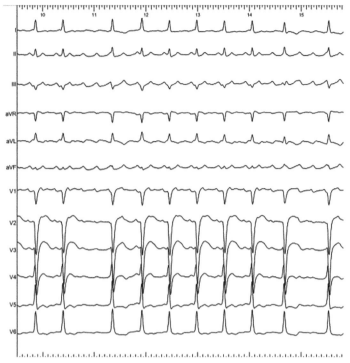

Fig. 7. AT, 12-lead ECG. Cycle length, 274 milliseconds; variation<5%.

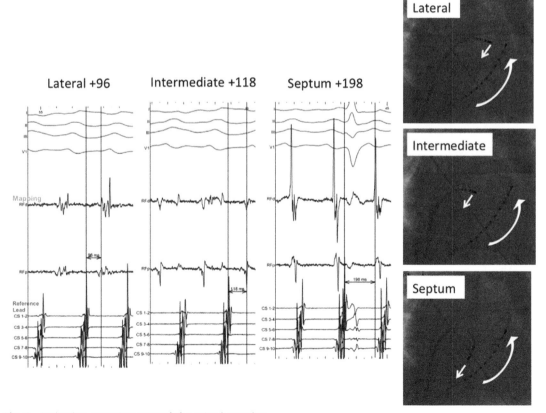

Fig. 8. Activation mapping around the mitral annulus.

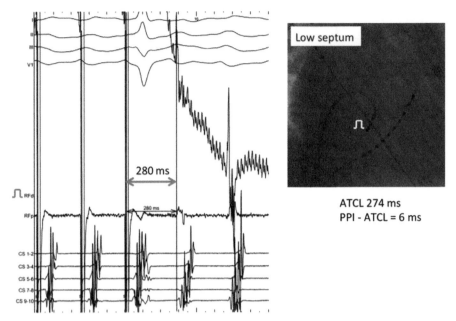

Fig. 9. Entrainment mapping at low septum.

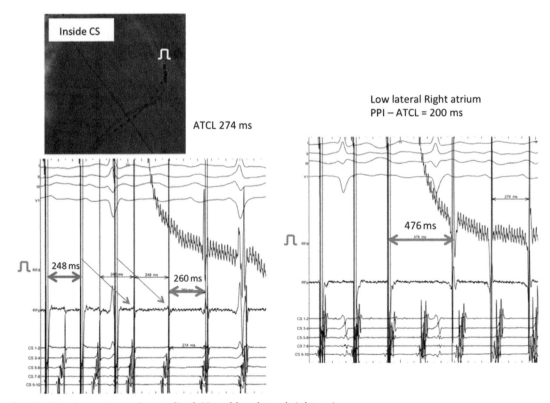

Fig. 10. Entrainment mapping at distal CS and low lateral right atrium.

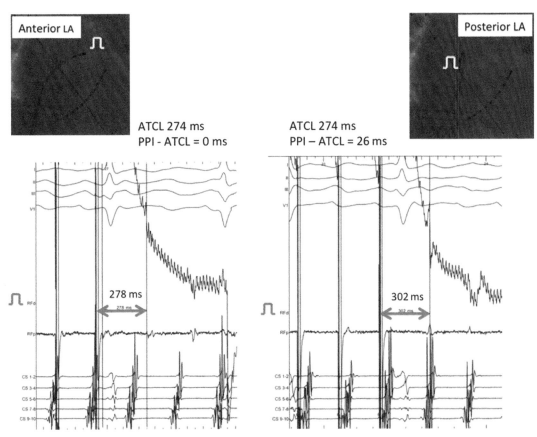

ATCL 274 ms
PPI - ATCL = 0 ms

ATCL 274 ms
PPI – ATCL = 26 ms

278 ms

302 ms

Fig. 11. Entrainment mapping at high lateral and posterior left atrium.

leaving 1 tachycardia looping around the mitral annulus. The activation and entrainment mapping confirmed counterclockwise perimitral flutter at 290 milliseconds.

At this stage, entrainment mapping from the posterior left atrium was repeated (**Fig. 14**) after conversion of double-loop tachycardia to perimitral flutter. The PPI minus TCL change, which

Counterclockwise Perimitral Flutter   +   Roof Dependent Flutter

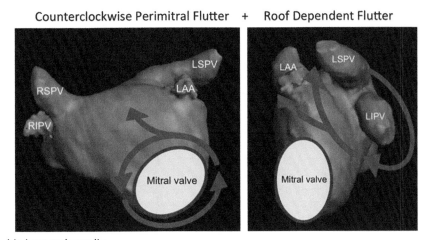

Fig. 12. Double-loop tachycardia.

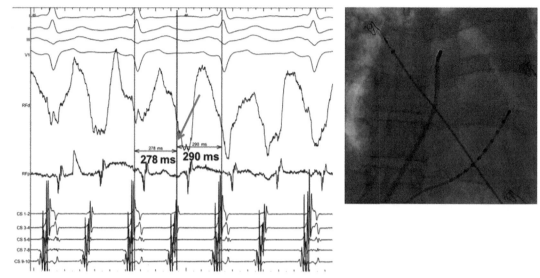

Fig. 13. Roof line ablation. ATCL prolonged to 290 milliseconds after 74 seconds of ablation on the roof.

was 26 milliseconds (see **Fig. 11**, right) during double-loop tachycardia, increased to 60 milliseconds during perimitral flutter, confirming the previous diagnosis of double-loop tachycardia.

INCARCERATED FOCAL AT

Fig. 15 shows a 12-lead ECG of a clinical AT at 308 milliseconds with beat-to-beat variation in cycle length less than 3%.[3]

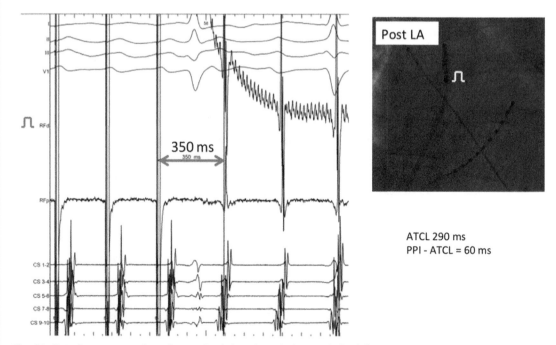

ATCL 290 ms
PPI - ATCL = 60 ms

Fig. 14. Entrainment mapping of posterior left atrium during perimitral flutter.

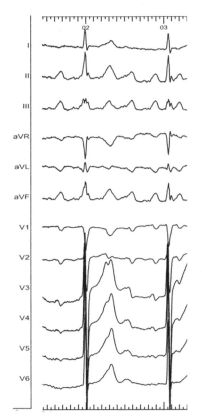

Fig. 15. AT, 12-lead ECG. Cycle length, 308 milliseconds; variation<3%.

Activation and entrainment mapping was consistent with diagnosis of focal-source AT from the base of the left atrial appendage. Ablation at the site of the earliest activity (at the base of the left appendage) resulted in conversion of stable tachycardia to unstable tachycardia without any change in the CS activation pattern, as shown in **Fig. 16**. The varying numbers represent changing beat-to-beat intervals during unstable tachycardia.

As shown in **Fig. 17**, the CS activation is out of phase with the activation of the left atrial appendage during unstable tachycardia. However, all the CS bipoles are activated in mutual tandem. Thus, there remains a possibility of 2 independent foci driving the unstable tachycardia (**Fig. 18**).

After successful termination of AT by focal ablation, sinus rhythm was restored in the atrial chamber but LAA continued to be in unstable AT, lending credence to the dual-foci hypothesis (see **Fig. 18**).

Fig. 19 shows the following:

1. The unstable tachycardia, confined to LAA, is mapped by repositioning the decapolar catheter inside the LAA to find its exact focal source, which could be lying inside the LAA.
2. Entrainment pacing at 310 milliseconds from the base of LAA reveals long return cycle length.
3. The bipoles 7-8 and 9-10 do not get entrained, which is revealed by beat-to-beat cycle length instability during entrainment.
4. During the return cycle, a long pause is noted on the entrained bipoles 1-2, 3-4, and 5-6, whereas unstable tachycardia continues on the nonentrained bipoles 7-8 and 9-10. This finding suggests that entrained bipoles lie away from the focal source. Also, the direction of activation of the bipoles of the decapolar catheter during unstable tachycardia is proximal to distal, suggesting an AT source lying close to bipole 9-10. Because bipoles 7-8 and 9-10 lie outside the LAA, it also confirms that the LAA is passively activated during unstable tachycardia.
5. During the maneuver, sinus rhythm continues in the atria.

With atria in sinus rhythm, the focal source of the clinical AT (CL - 308 milliseconds) was discovered in the region of bipole 9-10 (**Fig. 20**). This source lying in the left atrium was revealed after amplifying the signals multiple times the baseline value. After several previous attempts of focal-source ablation in and around the base of LAA, the conduction from the AT source (LA) to LAA occurred in 2:1 and 4:1 manner from base to apex of the LAA, as shown in **Fig. 20**, which proved that the LAA was a bystander for the focal-source AT arising from the anterior LA. From these findings, we concluded that the ablation of AT's exit site to the atria was responsible for restoration of SR with continuation of AT at the source. Also, the exit site to the LAA was different from the rest of the atria because tachycardia persisted in the LAA after restoration of sinus rhythm elsewhere.

LOCALIZED REENTRANT ATRIAL TACHYCARDIA MIMICKING MACROREENTRY

Fig. 21 shows clinical AT at 310 milliseconds with cycle length variation less than 5%.

As shown in **Fig. 22**, on the activation mapping, the anterior wall of the left atrium is activated simultaneously on the lateral and the septal sites. This finding ruled out perimitral flutter and right ATs. However, roof-dependent flutter could not be ruled in or out from the given information.

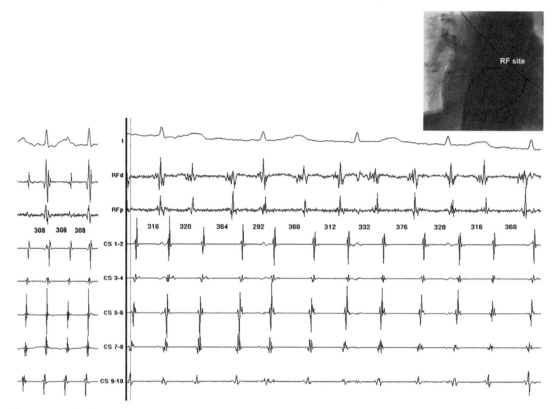

Fig. 16. Focal tachycardia: anterior left atrium conversion to unstable tachycardia during ablation.

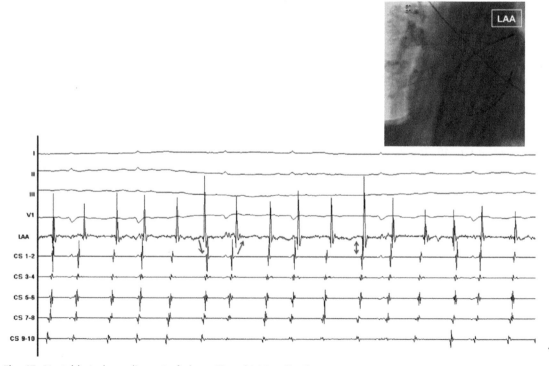

Fig. 17. Unstable tachycardia: out-of-phase CS and LAA activation.

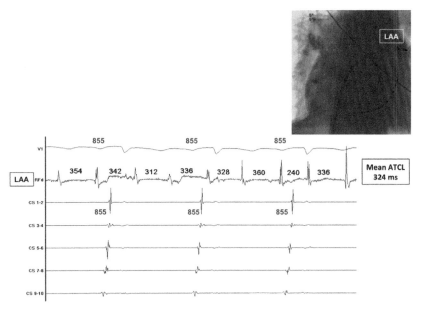

Fig. 18. After conversion to sinus rhythm.

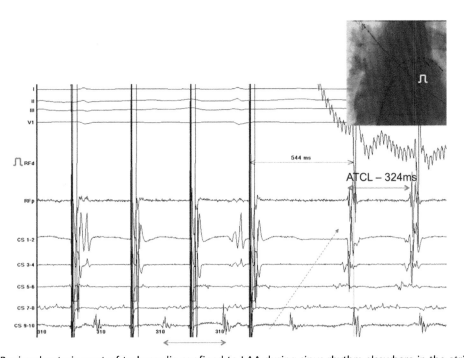

Fig. 19. Regional entrainment of tachycardia confined to LAA during sinus rhythm elsewhere in the atria.

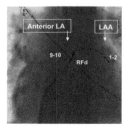

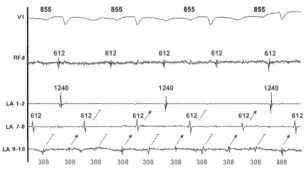

Fig. 20. Activation mapping of incarcerated tachycardia.

Further mapping of the left atrial anterior and posterior walls (**Figs. 23** and **24**), revealed an activation pattern consistent with roof-dependent flutter. Also, almost the entire cycle length of the AT was mapped.

The findings of entrainment mapping (**Fig. 25**) do not fit with the diagnosis of roof-dependent flutter, although the activation mapping suggests it. There is a trend toward shorter return cycle length from right to left, which suggests focal-source AT in the left atrium.

As shown in **Fig. 26**, a focal site on the high posterior left atrium showed highly fractionated and low-amplitude local signal spanning 60% of the AT cycle length. The local PPI minus ATCL change was 10 milliseconds. Put together, the findings of entrainment and activation mapping suggest localized reentry from this site. Ablation terminated the tachycardia and restored sinus rhythm after 70 seconds of radiofrequency application in this region. After restoration of sinus rhythm, the roof line was found to be blocked from the previous ablation procedure.

Important Points from Localized Reentry Mimicking Macroreentry

- Localized reentry near the blocked linear lesion can have an activation pattern mimicking macroreentry involving the site of linear lesion as a critical isthmus.
- Activation mapping may not provide a conclusive diagnosis even if the cycle length can be mapped in concurrence with macroreentry.
- Entrainment mapping is necessary to confirm the diagnostic possibility of macroreentry suggested by activation mapping.

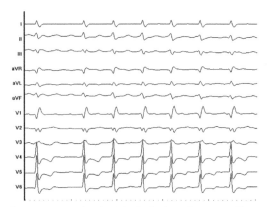

Fig. 21. AT, 12-lead ECG. Cycle length, 310 milliseconds; variation<5%.

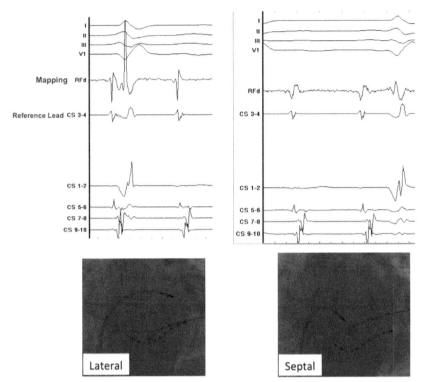

Fig. 22. Activation mapping, left atrium.

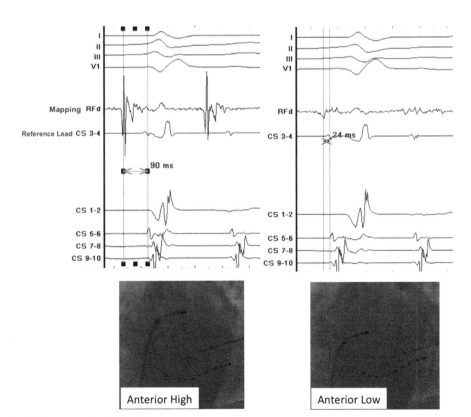

Fig. 23. Activation mapping, left atrium.

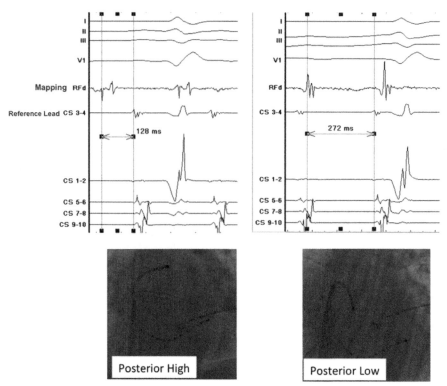

Fig. 24. Activation mapping, left atrium.

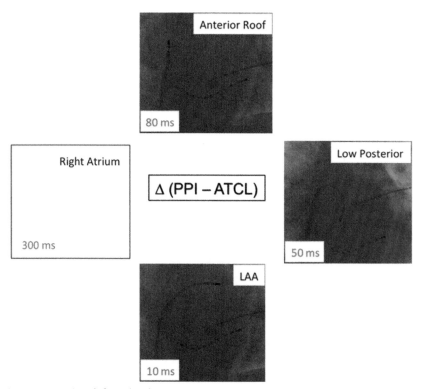

Fig. 25. Entrainment mapping, left and right atria.

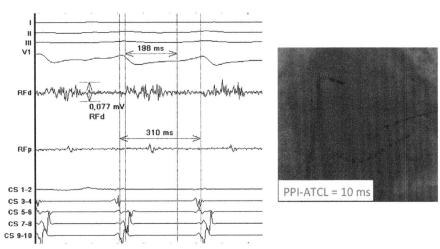

Fig. 26. Localization of the focal source: posterior left atrial roof.

REFERENCES

1. Miyazaki S, Shah AJ, Haïssaguerre M. Multiple atrial tachycardias after atrial fibrillation ablation: the importance of careful mapping and observation. Circ Arrhythm Electrophysiol 2011;4(2):251–4.

2. Matsuo S, Lim KT, Knecht S, et al. Dual independent atrial tachycardias after ablation of chronic atrial fibrillation. J Cardiovasc Electrophysiol 2008;19(9): 979–81.

3. Shah AJ, Wilton SB, Miyazaki S, et al. Restoration of sinus rhythm by incarceration, not elimination, of focal atrial tachycardia in left atrial substrate post atrial fibrillation ablation. Circ Arrhythm Electrophysiol 2011;4(3):e18–21.

Serial Atrial Tachycardias
Importance of Subtle Changes

Shinsuke Miyazaki, MD*, Ashok J. Shah, MD, Pierre Jais, MD

KEYWORDS

- Atrial tachycardia • Confined tachycardia • Multiple tachycardias • Catheter ablation

KEY POINTS

- Complex serial type of atrial tachycardias could be encountered in the context of atrial fibrillation ablation.
- Careful conventional mapping and precise interpretation of electrograms are required for the diagnosis and treatment.
- Subtle changes in electrogram could be a sign of transition of atrial tachycardia.
- A conduction delay in left atrial appendage should be checked after extensive ablation and/or multiple procedures to avoid its electrical isolation.

INTRODUCTION

Generally speaking, the mechanism of atrial tachycardias (ATs) after extensive atrial ablation and multiple ablation procedures is complex. It requires careful mapping and observation to reach a precise diagnosis. This article presents the mapping of ATs in two cases and highlights the subtle and complex characteristics that required careful mapping.

Case 1

A 47-year-old gentleman with an 8-year history of paroxysmal lone atrial fibrillation (AF), not controlled with amiodarone, was admitted with persistent AT for his third catheter ablation procedure.[1] At the first procedure, 7 years earlier, pulmonary vein (PV) isolation was performed. Six months earlier, reisolation of PVs, electrogram-based ablation, and linear ablation of left atrium (LA) roof and left mitral isthmus for inducible AT were performed, completely blocking both lines.

The AT cycle length (ATCL) was 275 ms during the start of the third procedure. No PV reconnection was observed. Mapping revealed the mechanism of clinical AT as a double loop reentry (see article elsewhere in this issue for further exploration of this topic) based on the finding that the activation sequence was compatible with both ATs and the Δpostpacing interval (PPI)-ATCL was less than 20 ms at LA roof, anterior and posterior LA, as well as at the mitral annulus. After 74 seconds of radiofrequency ablation catheter (RF) application on the LA roof, clinical AT was converted to perimitral AT with a cycle length of 290 ms (**Fig. 1**). The morphology of the P wave (**Fig. 2**) and the activation sequence of the coronary sinus (CS) electrograms did not change (see **Fig. 1**). Following endocardial and epicardial RF application on the left mitral isthmus, the second AT got converted to the third AT (**Figs. 3** and **4**). However, there was no change in the ATCL or the activation sequence of the CS electrograms (see **Fig. 3**). The conversion was marked by a change in the morphology of the P wave (see **Fig. 4**). The third AT was diagnosed as focal AT originating from the high LA septum, and 9 seconds of RF

Conflicts of Interest: None.
Disclosures: None.
Department of Rhythmologie, The Hôpital Cardiologique du Haut-Lévêque and the Université Victor Segalen Bordeaux II, Bordeaux, France
* Corresponding author. Hôpital Haut Lévêque, 33604 Bordeaux-Pessac, France.
E-mail address: mshinsuke@k3.dion.ne.jp

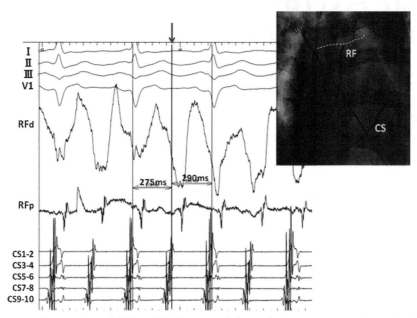

Fig. 1. The moment of conversion of AT1 to AT2. Fluoroscopic image in the anteroposterior projection shows the catheter position during roof line ablation. The application prolongs the cycle length from 275 ms to 290 ms (*red arrow*); however, the coronary sinus (CS) activation sequence did not change. d, distal electrode pair; p, proximal electrode pair; RF, radiofrequency ablation catheter. (*Adapted from* Miyazaki S, Shah AJ, Haïssaguerre M. Multiple atrial tachycardias after atrial fibrillation ablation: the importance of careful mapping and observation. Circ Arrhythm Electrophysiol 2011;4:251–4; with permission.)

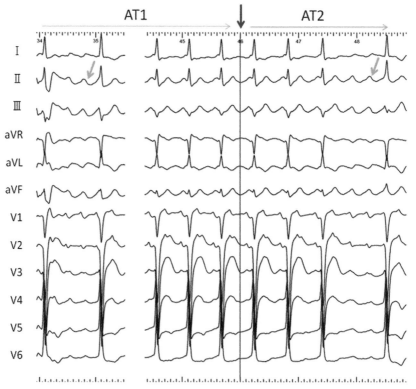

Fig. 2. P-wave morphology unchanged (*green arrow*) during the transition (*red line*) of AT. (*Adapted from* Miyazaki S, Shah AJ, Haïssaguerre M. Multiple atrial tachycardias after atrial fibrillation ablation: the importance of careful mapping and observation. Circ Arrhythm Electrophysiol 2011;4:251–4; with permission.)

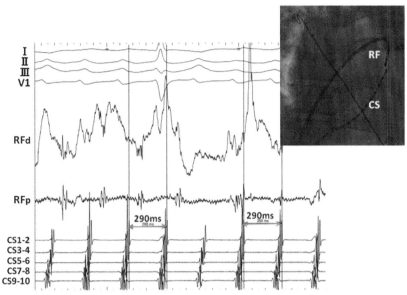

Fig. 3. The moment of conversion of AT2 to AT3. Fluoroscopic image in the anteroposterior projection shows the catheter position during mitral isthmus line ablation. Coronary sinus (CS) activation sequence and cycle length unchanged. (*Adapted from* Miyazaki S, Shah AJ, Haïssaguerre M. Multiple atrial tachycardias after atrial fibrillation ablation: the importance of careful mapping and observation. Circ Arrhythm Electrophysiol 2011;4:251–4; with permission.)

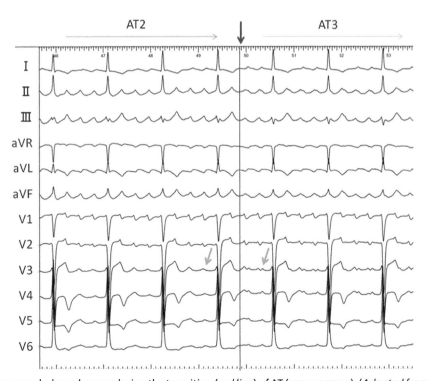

Fig. 4. P-wave morphology changes during the transition (*red line*) of AT (*green arrows*). (*Adapted from* Miyazaki S, Shah AJ, Haïssaguerre M. Multiple atrial tachycardias after atrial fibrillation ablation: the importance of careful mapping and observation. Circ Arrhythm Electrophysiol 2011;4:251–4; with permission.)

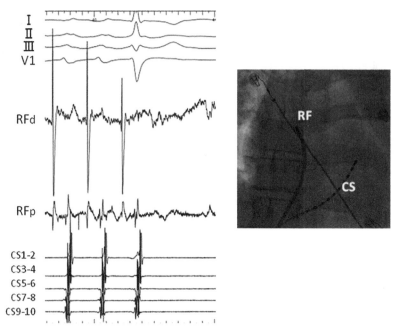

Fig. 5. AT terminates following 9 seconds of application at LA high septum. (*Adapted from* Miyazaki S, Shah AJ, Haïssaguerre M. Multiple atrial tachycardias after atrial fibrillation ablation: the importance of careful mapping and observation. Circ Arrhythm Electrophysiol 2011;4:251–4; with permission.)

application at this site restored sinus rhythm (**Fig. 5**). PPI mapping was used to localize this focus; ΔPPI-ATCL was longer at left middle septum, fossa ovalis, right septum, and CS ostium than at the left high septum. However, it was 0 at

the site of successful ablation (**Fig. 6**). After the confirmation of bidirectional block across the left mitral isthmus, the LA roof, and the cavotricuspid isthmus lines using differential pacing techniques, the fourth AT was easily induced by proximal CS

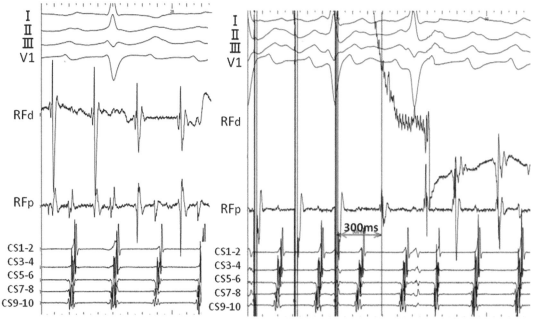

Fig. 6. Activation mapping (*left*) and entrainment mapping (*right*) show that the origin of AT3 was high septum. (*Adapted from* Miyazaki S, Shah AJ, Haïssaguerre M. Multiple atrial tachycardias after atrial fibrillation ablation: the importance of careful mapping and observation. Circ Arrhythm Electrophysiol 2011;4:251–4; with permission.)

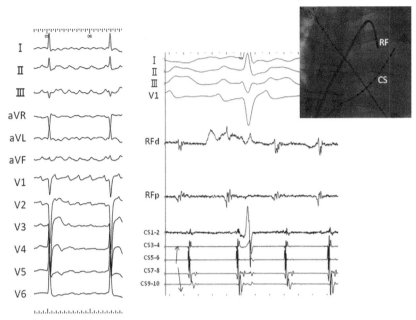

Fig. 7. 12-Lead ECG of AT4 did not show isoelectric line. CS activation sequence shows eccentric activation with earliest activation of bipole CS5-6 (*red arrows*). It is eliminated after 15 seconds of RF application in the postero-lateral LA. (*Adapted from* Miyazaki S, Shah AJ, Haïssaguerre M. Multiple atrial tachycardias after atrial fibrillation ablation: the importance of careful mapping and observation. Circ Arrhythm Electrophysiol 2011;4:251–4; with permission.)

burst pacing at 250 ms (**Fig. 7**). It was diagnosed as focal AT originating from the posterolateral LA below and behind the left mitral isthmus line of block. It was eliminated by 15 seconds of RF

application and termination was marked by the activation of bipole CS1-2 in the absence of activation of the remainder of the CS bipoles (see **Fig. 7**; **Fig. 8**). PPI mapping was used to localize this

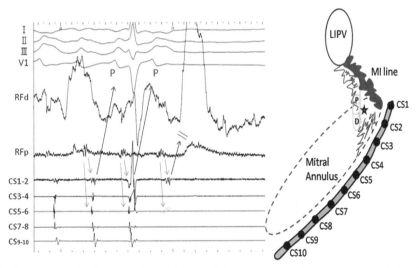

Fig. 8. Final tachycardia beat activates only distal CS, and does not generate P wave (*arrows*). Possible explanation for the observed phenomenon (*right*). The focus (*violet star*) is below the complete MI line (*dense red line*) and is surrounded by the scar (*shaggy red line*) due to previous MI ablation. The application closes the exit closest to the focus, and the final beat activates the small closed MI area. MI, mitral isthmus. (*Adapted from* Miyazaki S, Shah AJ, Haïssaguerre M. Multiple atrial tachycardias after atrial fibrillation ablation: the importance of careful mapping and observation. Circ Arrhythm Electrophysiol 2011;4:251–4; with permission.)

focus, and ΔPPI-ATCL was 0 at this site. No tachycardia was inducible on further testing.

This case demonstrates four different ATs, including two macroreentrant and two focal ATs, in a patient who was previously subjected to extensive LA ablation procedure. The first and second ATs were macroreentrant ATs, which were diagnosed with activation and entrainment mapping. Conversion from the first AT to the second one was identified just by the prolongation in ATCL. Possible explanation of this change is that because CS activation was mostly determined by the perimitral component of the first AT, it did not change during its conversion to the second AT, which was an isolated perimitral AT with longer ATCL than the previous AT. P-wave morphology did not change. Theoretically, after extensive LA ablation, the relative contribution of the LA toward the composition of the surface P wave should be smaller compared with that of the RA. In other words, RA activation should be predominantly responsible for determining the

morphology of the surface P wave. This observation was confirmed later during the sinus rhythm. Conversion of first AT to the second one did not result in any change in the activation pattern of the RA, the passive chamber, which could explain the absence of alteration in the morphology of the P wave between the two ATs. The third AT was identified as a focal AT. Interestingly, the CS activation sequence and the ATCL did not change when macroreentrant AT was converted to focal AT and the conversion was identified only by a subtle change in the P-wave morphology. Because the focus lay on the left side of the high septum and the mitral isthmus line was completely blocked during ablation of the second AT, it seemed that any change in the activation sequence of the CS was forbidden. Although the conversion of second AT to the third one involved a subtle change, careful observation of the P-wave morphology helped to clinch the diagnosis. The fourth AT could be quickly identified as focal AT because bidirectional block across all the lines

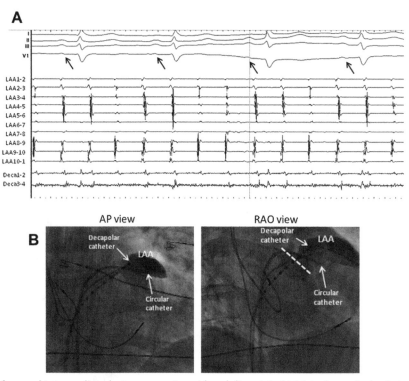

Fig. 9. (A) Surface and intracardiac electrograms. A rapid and dissociated LAA tachycardia (cycle length: 250 ms) surrounded by atria in sinus rhythm (cycle length: 850 ms) is evident on intracardiac recordings. The arrows show sinus P waves. Note that the distal part of the decapolar catheter is placed in the LAA. (B) Contrast angiography of LAA. The circular mapping catheter was in the LAA and the decapolar catheter at the anterior LA with the distal portion in the LAA. The LAA anatomy was normal. The dotted line approximately delineates the area in which the tachycardia is confined. LAA, LA appendage. (*Adapted from* Miyazaki S, Nault I, Jaïs P, et al. Atrial tachycardia confined within the left atrial appendage. J Cardiovasc Electrophysiol 2010;21:933–5; with permission.)

was established just a short while earlier, which obviated macroreentrant ATs. Because the CS activation pattern during the fourth AT was such that the earliest activation occurred at bipole CS5-6, mapping around it confirmed low postero-lateral LA as the source of this AT. In this case, to identify the focus, not only the activation mapping but also the PPI mapping was very useful. The authors performed PPI mapping several times from both sides of the atrial septum to precisely spot the third AT. The interesting part of the fourth AT was its mode of termination. The last tachy-cardia beat resulted in activation of a small area of the LA around the proximal electrode pair of the ablation catheter and the bipole CS1-2. Tachy-cardia terminated without activation of any of the remaining CS bipoles and inscription of the P wave on the surface ECG. A possible

explanation for the observed phenomenon could be that the RF application closed the exit of impulse to the proximal CS bipoles from the focus, which was surrounded by the ablation lesions in the near vicinity, a blocked mitral isthmus laterally, and a blocked roof line superiorly. The last beat of the tachycardia did not activate the proximal CS, which was along the route of impulse traveling to the RA. Because the activation of RA was mainly responsible for the inscription of the P wave on the surface ECG, it is possible that because the tachycardia terminated without the activation of RA, there was an absence of P wave (see **Fig. 8**). The relation between the P wave and the RA acti-vation was supported by the findings during sinus rhythm. The most part of the sinus P wave coin-cided with the activation of the RA, and the activa-tion of CS was found to be delayed suggestive of

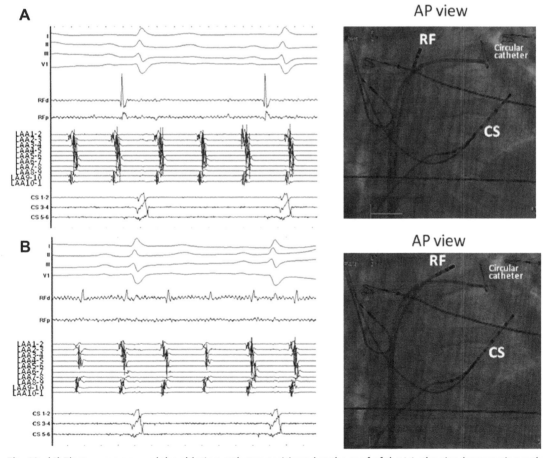

Fig. 10. (*A*) Electrograms record the ablation catheter positioned at the roof of the LA, the circular mapping cath-eter positioned in the LAA, and the decapolar catheter inside the CS. (*B*) Electrograms are recorded by the abla-tion catheter positioned at the anterior LA near the LAA, the circular mapping catheter positioned in the LAA, and the decapolar catheter inside CS. The tachycardia is confined within the LAA and on the anterior LA wall near the LAA. (*Adapted from* Miyazaki S, Nault I, Jaïs P, et al. Atrial tachycardia confined within the left atrial appendage. J Cardiovasc Electrophysiol 2010;21:933–5; with permission.)

huge interatrial conduction delay due to extensive ablation.

A previous report demonstrated that the presence of isoelectric interval between the tachycardia P waves may be useful in making the diagnosis of a focal mechanism of tachycardia.[2] In other words, macroreentrant circuits lack an isoelectric interval and AT with a nonreentrant mechanism presents with discrete P waves separated by an isoelectric interval on the ECG. However, this holds true in the patients without extensive atrial tissue ablation. The authors believe that large conduction delay due to extensive ablation could make the focal AT lose an isoelectric interval on the ECG, as observed in this case. On the contrary, extensive atrial ablation is also responsible for very slow conduction spanning over a large part of tachycardia cycle length but occurring in a small part of the macroreentrant circuit. Such a long delay can inscribe an isoelectric interval in between the macroreentrant-tachycardia P waves on ECG, which may not be sensitive enough to record slow activation occurring in a small area of the atrium.

Case 2

A 72-year-old man was referred for catheter ablation of symptomatic and persistent AF lasting 3 months.[3] AF was refractory to pharmacologic therapy and recurred shortly after each electrical cardioversion. He had sick sinus syndrome for which a dual-chamber pacemaker was implanted.

The baseline AF cycle length measured in the LA appendage (LAA) was 183 ms. The four PVs were isolated, electrogram-based LA ablation was undertaken, and LA roof and mitral isthmus lines were deployed, resulting in AFs conversion to AT. However, frequent changes were observed in LA activation suggesting multiple ATs. Sinus rhythm was restored 25 minutes after intravenous infusion of 300 mg of amiodarone.

Following restoration of sinus rhythm, the RF catheter was brought inside the LAA to assess conduction block along the LA lines and a rapid and regular activity was observed. The LAA tachycardia had a cycle length of 250 ms (**Fig. 9**). Further detailed mapping of both atria recorded normal sinus rhythm in the CS and in all parts of right and left atria except inside the LAA and

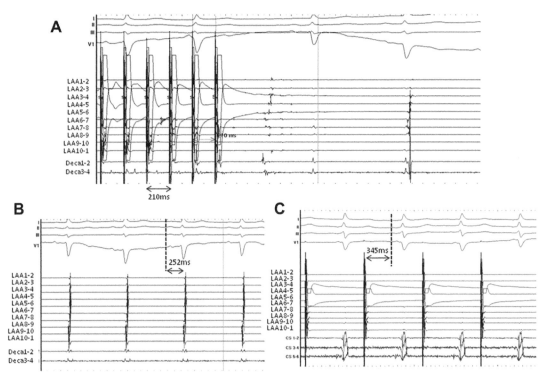

Fig. 11. (A) LAA overdrive pacing terminates the local tachycardia. (B) After termination of local tachycardia, LA-LAA conduction is significantly delayed during sinus rhythm (252 ms from the onset of P wave to LAA) and (C) during pacing from the LAA (345 ms from pacing spike to the onset of P wave). (*Adapted from* Miyazaki S, Nault I, Jaïs P, et al. Atrial tachycardia confined within the left atrial appendage. J Cardiovasc Electrophysiol 2010;21:933–5; with permission.)

a collar of anterior LA wall near the LAA (**Fig. 10**). An angiography of the LAA was performed and fluttering LAA activity and LAA emptying were observed (see **Fig. 9**B). Complete LA roof line and mitral isthmus line blocks were documented by differential pacing technique.

The tachycardia was then terminated by a local burst pacing at 210 ms in the LAA (**Fig. 11**A) and further ectopic beats or reinitiation were not observed. The LA-LAA conduction was examined during sinus rhythm by pacing in the LA and LAA and bidirectional conduction was observed between both structures. A significant conduction delay (252 ms from the onset of P wave to LAA) was observed during sinus rhythm (see **Fig. 11**B) and LAA-LA conduction was observed during LAA pacing at pacing cycle length 700 ms or longer (see **Fig. 11**C). The dissociation observed during LAA tachycardia could, therefore, be attributed to a rate-dependent concealed conduction.

Isolated focal source from the CS and the LA were reported after ablation providing further evidence for the existence of such sources.[4] Moreover, the LAA was one of the preferential locations for localized reentrant circuits in patients developing left AT following AF catheter-ablation. In this case, the local tachycardia continued independently for more than 20 minutes, at a stable cycle length. The electrically isolated area consisted of the LAA and the anterior LA in its vicinity, which was surrounded by atrial tissue in sinus rhythm. After termination of the isolated tachycardia, the conduction between the LA and the LAA was unmasked despite the isolation during LAA tachycardia. Pacing from LA and LAA revealed conduction with a significant activation delay between the two structures, suggesting that the conduction between LA and LAA was rate-dependent. This altered conduction could be attributable to a combination of anterior LA scar due to LA ablation, mitral isthmus line block, and to the electrophysiologic pharmacodynamics of amiodarone. Such alteration in conduction may be deleterious for atrial transport function. Therefore, no attempt to reinduce the arrhythmia and no further ablation were performed because further ablation could have resulted in complete isolation of the LAA. Extensive LA ablation could yield electrical isolation of the LAA and, therefore, mechanical paralysis of LAA, potentially leading to an increased risk of clot formation within it. Although the reconduction was observed during follow-up in most of the cases with initial LAA isolation, careful monitoring seems to be necessary during extensive LA ablation to avoid the risk of LAA isolation. This case proves that the LAA is capable of sustaining AT independently from the LA and can, therefore, represent an active source in the genesis and maintenance of AF.

REFERENCES

1. Miyazaki S, Shah AJ, Haïssaguerre M. Multiple atrial tachycardias after atrial fibrillation ablation: the importance of careful mapping and observation. Circ Arrhythm Electrophysiol 2011;4:251–4.

2. Shah D, Sunthorn H, Burri H, et al. Narrow, slow-conducting isthmus dependent left atrial reentry developing after ablation for atrial fibrillation: ECG characterisation and elimination by focal RF ablation. J Cardiovasc Electrophysiol 2006;17:508–15.

3. Miyazaki S, Nault I, Jaïs P, et al. Atrial tachycardia confined within the left atrial appendage. J Cardiovasc Electrophysiol 2010;21:933–5.

4. Knecht S, O'Neill MD, Matsuo S, et al. Focal arrhythmia confined within the coronary sinus and maintaining atrial fibrillation. J Cardiovasc Electrophysiol 2007;18:1140–6.

Advent of Noninvasive Mapping of Atrial Tachycardias

Ashok J. Shah, MD*, Meleze Hocini, MD, Pierre Jais, MD,
Michel Haissaguerre, MD

KEYWORDS

- Noninvasive map • Unipolar electrogram • Atrial tachycardia

KEY POINTS

- Our experience with a novel, noninvasive, mapping system in a wide range of patients with and without previous ablation demonstrates the feasibility of accurately identifying the atria where the atrial tachycardia (AT) is located and defining the AT mechanism.
- Recently developed algorithms based on regional and global atrial activation patterns combined with tissue level information such as local electrogram morphology and voltage have successfully helped overcome previous diagnostic limitations and improved the usefulness of the system in the noninvasive diagnosis of even the most complex forms of clinical atrial tachycardias.

INTRODUCTION

For more than 100 years, 12-lead electrocardiography (ECG) has been the standard-of-care, noninvasive tool providing vital electrical information from limited sites on the chest to diagnose a cardiac disorder, its possible mechanism, and the likely site of origin. Advances in noninvasive imaging technology have yielded tools such as computed tomography (CT), magnetic resonance imaging (MRI), and positron emission tomography (PET); these and several other tools have provided novel insights into the clinical physiology, anatomy, and pathologies. These noninvasive diagnostic methods have also improved patient care by providing valuable guidance in the therapeutic management of several cardiac and noncardiac disorders, and many of them have replaced the invasive imaging techniques as gold standards.

In cardiac electrophysiology and arrhythmias, several decades of research have led to the development of high-resolution body-surface mapping, a novel three-dimensional (3D), noninvasive, cardiac mapping and imaging modality. The team of Yoram Rudy (Cardiac Bioelectricity and Arrhythmia Center, Washington University, St. Louis, MO, USA) has been particularly active in the development of this novel tool for more than 2 decades. This technique images potentials, electrograms, and activation sequences (isochrones) on the epicardial surface of the heart. This tool has been investigated in normal cardiac electrophysiology and various tachyarrhythmic, interventricular conduction, and anomalous depo-repolarization disorders. It is emerging as a tool of substantially greater clinical value than the 12-lead ECG in the diagnostic and therapeutic management of cardiac rhythm disorders.

In this article, the experience of the authors in mapping atrial tachycardia (AT) using this noninvasive 3D electroanatomic system is described, followed by clinical illustrations of noninvasively mapped ATs correlated with the invasive diagnosis.

Conflicts of Interest: None.
Disclosures: Ashok J Shah is a paid consultant to Meleze Hocini, Pierre Jais and Michel Haissaguerre are stock owners in CardioInsight Inc, Cleveland, Ohio, USA.
Hôpital Cardiologique du Haut-Lévêque, Department of Rhythmologie, Avenue de Magellan, Bordeaux-Pessac 33604, France
* Corresponding author. Hôpital Haut Lévêque, Bordeaux, Pessac 33604, France.
E-mail address: drashahep@gmail.com

NONINVASIVE AT MAPPING EXPERIENCE
Methods

In a systematic comparative study, noninvasive electrocardiomapping (ECM) (CardioInsight Inc, Cleveland, OH, USA) was undertaken before an invasive electrophysiology (EP) study and ablation of clinical AT.[1] The accuracy of the system in diagnosing the arrhythmia mechanism and the location of the arrhythmia in centrifugal (focal) AT was determined by comparison with invasive maps (fluoroscopy-based with or without Carto or NavX) and confirmed by successful ablation. Each map consisted of a patient-specific 3D biatrial anatomy obtained from noncontrast CT scan.

Electrocardiographic mapping

The mathematical principles underlying the computational methods and the techniques used in the construction of electrocardiomaps using multiple body-surface electrodes have been previously described.[2–4] The procedure undertaken in a clinical setup to obtain noninvasive maps using the ECM system is described briefly. A 252-electrode disposable vest is applied to the patient's torso and connected to the ECM system to record the unipolar potentials. These potentials constitute the field. A noncontrast thoracic CT scan is then performed to obtain high-resolution images of the heart and the vest electrodes. The position of the electrodes relative to the reconstructed 3D epicardial biatrial geometry is obtained via segmentation of the CT images. The system reconstructs epicardial unipolar electrograms from the field using mathematical reconstruction algorithms. These reconstructed potentials constitute the source. Activation maps are computed using a traditional, unipolar electrogram, intrinsic deflection-based ($-dV/dT_{max}$) method. In addition, a novel directional activation map using electrogram morphology and local propagation between adjacent electrograms facilitates analysis of the ECM. Signal averaging of tachycardia P waves (field) during long RR intervals helps to improve the signal quality.

All ECMaps are analyzed in a stepwise manner as follows:

1. A window of 1 or more tachycardia cycles involving distinct tachycardia P wave(s) and/or the tachycardia-initiating beat, if available, is selected starting with the predominant deflection on the field signal.
2. The source electrical activity is analyzed such that the negative electrogram morphology (QS or Qr) represents an active chamber among the 2 atria and positive morphology (R or Rs) identifies the passively activated atrium.
3. The maps provide biatrial activation patterns during tachycardia, which can help diagnose the mechanism of AT. The AT is broadly divided into centrifugal (focal source) and macroreentrant. Macroreentrant AT includes perimitral, cavotricuspid isthmus-dependent and roof-dependent AT. In centrifugal ATs, the location of the arrhythmia source is determined. The definition of macroreentrant and focal ATs is based on the statement from a joint expert group from the Working Group of Arrhythmias of the European Society of Cardiology and the North American Society of Pacing and Electrophysiology.[5] An activation map of macroreentry encompasses more than 75% of the AT cycle length spread over 3 or more distinct atrial segments in a reentrant fashion around a large central obstacle. In focal ATs, global atrial activation occurs centrifugally from a small source (focus).

Validation by invasive EP

All clinical ATs were first mapped at the bedside using the ECM system, followed by subsequent invasive mapping and ablation. Fluoroscopy and an intracardiac, electrogram-based, conventional approach was used to validate the ECM diagnosis. 3D electroanatomic mapping systems (Carto or NavX) aided validation of the activation pattern of macroreentrant AT and the location of centrifugal AT was diagnosed noninvasively. The confirmation of the diagnosis was obtained when ablation of the target site/linear lesion resulted in successful termination of AT.

Results

Among the study population (n = 52, 1 clinical AT per patient), structural heart disease was present in 18 (35%) and 2 patients had undergone bilateral lung transplantation. The atrial fibrillation (AF) ablation procedure was undertaken previously in 27 (52%) patients (including surgical ablation in 1 patient). The mean cycle length of the clinical AT was 284 ± 85 milliseconds. The ECM diagnosis was evaluable in 48 patients in whom an invasive EP diagnosis was confirmed by successful ablation. In the remaining 4 patients, clinical AT converted to another rhythm (AT/AF/sinus) before invasive mapping was completed, and therefore, these patients were excluded from the comparative analysis.

Comparison of diagnostic maps (ECM vs EP)

Of 48 ATs, 27 were diagnosed invasively as macroreentrant (18 cavotricuspid isthmus-dependent, 5 perimitral and 3 roof-dependent) ATs including 1 AT around the right atrial postatriotomy scar and 21 as centrifugal arrhythmias (15 from the left atrium, 4 from the right, and 2 from interatrial septum). All were successfully terminated by ablation to the sinus rhythm in 44 patients or another AT in 4 patients. ECM accurately diagnosed 85% (23/27) of the macroreentrant ATs and 100% (21/21) of the centrifugal ATs. Overall, ECM identified the mechanism of AT as macroreentrant versus centrifugal activation including localization of the focal source in 92% (44/48) patients.

Previous AF ablation and accuracy of ECM

The diagnostic accuracy of ECM in patients with previous AF ablation was 83% (19/23 ATs). In the remaining 25 patients without any previous atrial ablation, the diagnosis was accurately obtained in 25/25 ATs (100%).

Discussion

This study demonstrates the clinical usefulness of an external, single-beat, 3D mapping system for mapping simple and complex ATs. The overall diagnostic accuracy of ECM compared with EP, the invasive gold standard, was 92% (100% in patients with de novo AT and 83% in patients with previous AF ablations). ECM was particularly useful and adept at accurately diagnosing 100% centrifugal ATs including 13 (62%) ATs in patients with previous AF ablation. Among centrifugal ATs, differentiation of true focal from localized (not macro) reentrant AT could not be established. Although such differentiation is important from a mechanistic perspective, it does not alter the target for ablation.[6]

Initially, it was challenging to map perimitral AT (the first 4 cases of perimitral AT could not be diagnosed) noninvasively. The primary reasons for failure were (1) 2:1 atrioventricular conduction, precluding selection of a full tachycardia cycle (unmasked by the QRST complex) and (2) a low signal to noise ratio from low voltage electrograms along most of the perimitral circuit as a result of extensive previous ablation. Noise reduction using a signal averaging algorithm is practical and clinically useful for stable monomorphic arrhythmias without altering the morphology or frequency content of low-amplitude signals by traditional filtering techniques. In these patients, signal averaging could not be used because the QRST complex obscured the P waves. Signal processing techniques to stop the ventricular complex from obscuring the P waves warrants further development. Alternatively, administration of atrioventricular node blockers or simple pacing maneuvers during the invasive procedure could have been undertaken to unmask 1 or more P waves (ie, a postventricular pacing pause in the R-R interval

can unobscure P wave(s) from the QRST complex and allow capture of multiple AT cycles.)

Limitations

1. A current limitation of arrhythmia mapping using this system is its inability to directly map the septum because it is not included or displayed on the cardiac surface geometry. However, a septal source can be deduced by analyzing the location (interatrial groove) and timing of the epicardial breakthrough.
2. ECM is considered to provide epicardial biatrial maps. Although there is experimental evidence for differential activation of the contiguous endoepicardium in at least some parts of the atria, the difference may be considered negligible in this multicenter study; there was virtually no difference between the epicardial ECMap and endocardial targets of ablation as seen in previously published reports.[7,8] Moreover, the atrial tissue is much thinner (in most parts) than the ventricular myocardium and although we did not evaluate the quantitative resolution of the system in this study, the clinical target was observed to be within 1 cm of the actual ablation site.
3. ATs with a small-amplitude field (P waves) are challenging to analyze. The amplitude of the tachycardia P wave depends on the rate and direction of the wavefront activating/depolarizing the local site and the amount of myocardial fibers recruited per unit time in the process. The local edema generated from ongoing ablation in the region can affect both invasive/noninvasive electrogram recording and local ablation. Further developments in signal processing techniques will help improve the accuracy of diagnosis using low-amplitude signals.

Clinical Perspectives and Current Progress

1. ECM can noninvasively provide global atrial activation patterns of sustained as well as transient AT from a single tachycardia beat/cycle, whereas the sequential beat mapping technique requires sustained AT or repetitive occurrence of ectopic beats. Single-beat simultaneous mapping can be crucial when the clinical AT changes frequently from one form to another and for mapping the beats that trigger sustained arrhythmias such as AF. Such a beat-to-beat analysis allows tracking of the changes, which may arise spontaneously or after ablation. ECM is a noninvasive system and can therefore be applied at the bedside, potentially providing the EP physician with a lot more data to plan the ablation procedure.

2. ECM provides further advantages over conventional ECG by enhancing the usefulness of the current system for organized arrhythmias allowing noninvasive visualization of the path of the macroreentrant circuit. In patients with extensive ablation, the ECG pattern of tachycardia P waves often loses its classic appearance, thereby misleading the diagnostic exercise. In this group of patients, ECM helps us to understand how and why the ECG fails to show the classic P wave patterns of certain arrhythmias such as common flutter and focal ATs.

3. With our experience in noninvasive atrial tachycardia mapping using algorithms based on regional and global atrial activation patterns and incorporating tissue level information such as local electrograms (ie, morphology) and voltage, we have been successful in overcoming the previous limitation (ie, diagnosis of perimitral AT) encountered in the earlier study. The diagnosis of several different reentrant and focal ATs, including perimitral and double-loop (roof-dependent + perimitral) ATs in patients with previous AF ablation or ongoing AT/AF ablation has been successfully accomplished both at the bedside and perprocedurally.

4. Real-time panoramic mapping, progress in computer technology, and new signal processing techniques have extended the use of a noninvasive diagnostic system beyond organized arrhythmia to fibrillatory rhythms of the cardiac chamber. Such a system is capable of providing a roadmap consisting of limited targets (sources) of ablation in persistent AF.

ILLUSTRATED CLINICAL CASES

Clinical Case 1

In a 76-year-old woman with 14-year history of AF, 2 attempts at cardioversion assisted by oral amiodarone therapy failed to maintain sinus rhythm. Radiofrequency ablation was recommended for her persistent (3 months) AF resulting in severe secondary cardiomyopathy. On continued amiodarone therapy before ablation, AF intermittently organized into varying morphologies of transient AT. On the day of the EP procedure, noninvasive mapping was undertaken perprocedurally. **Figs. 1** and **2** show the presenting rhythm on 12-lead ECG (AT at 280 milliseconds) and the corresponding ECM, respectively. The AT was mapped invasively using the point-by-point mapping technique and confirmed by entrainment mapping as a cavotricuspid isthmus–dependent counterclockwise flutter in concordance with the noninvasive 3D map.

Clinical Case 2

In a patient with nonobstructive hypertrophic cardiomyopathy and 2 previous ablations for persistent AF, the presenting rhythm was AT at

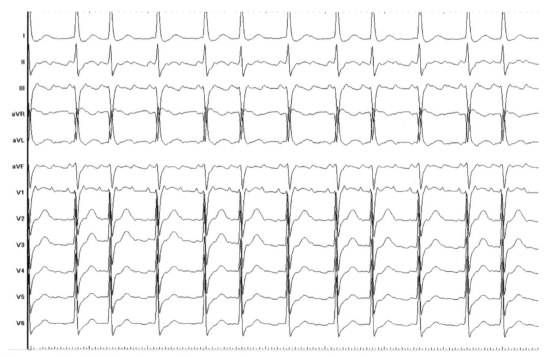

Fig. 1. A 12-lead-ECG for a 76-year-old woman with persistent AF of 3 months duration shows amiodarone organized rhythm (AT at 280 milliseconds) at the start of the procedure.

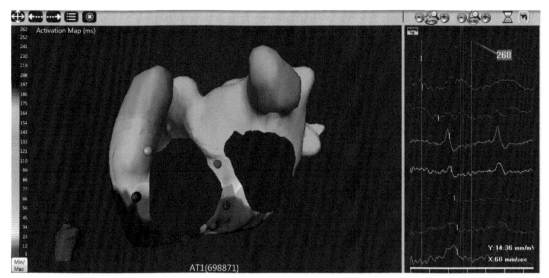

Fig. 2. An isochronal electrocardiomap of the AT (cycle length 280 milliseconds) shown in **Fig. 1** is diagnostic of counterclockwise peritricuspid AT. The color-coded time scale is seen on the left and the local unipolar electrograms during 2 AT cycles are displayed on the right. The color of the electrogram corresponds to the site of the same colored spot on the biatrial geometry. The –dV/dT markers are shown as short vertical white lines on each unipolar electrogram.

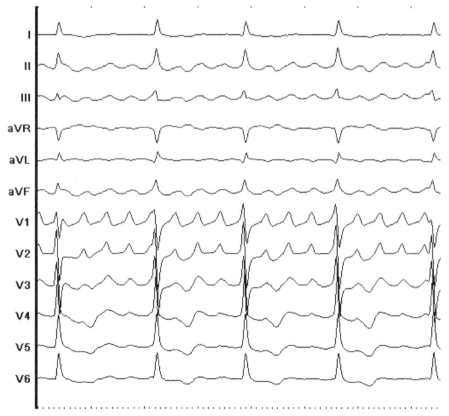

Fig. 3. A 12-lead-ECG for a patient with nonobstructive hypertrophic cardiomyopathy and 2 previous ablations for persistent AF. The presenting rhythm was AT at 226 milliseconds at the start of the third ablation procedure.

ECM – Focal-source from Roof

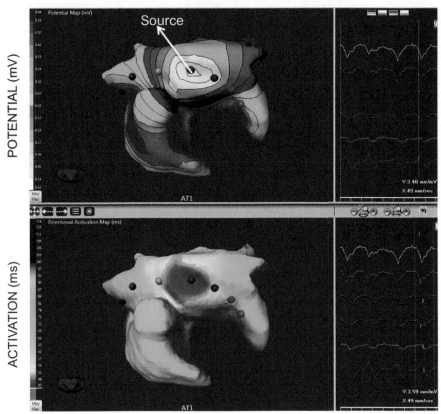

Fig. 4. (*Top*) The perprocedural noninvasive isopotential ECMap at time 0 seconds shows the focal source AT (at 226 milliseconds) emerging from the left atrial roof. The isopotential map assigns the most negative (<0) potential value (in millivolts) to the site with the earliest depolarization in the selected window of the AT cycle length. The potential values are color coded. The colors change from white to yellow to orange in decreasing order of negativity. Values greater than 0 (positive potential) are presented in shades of green in increasing order of positivity (*light to dark*). This map is a snapshot of the onset of depolarization (*white*) on the left atrial roof. The corresponding local unipolar electrograms during more than 3 AT cycles are displayed on the right. (*Bottom*) The corresponding isochronal map. The –dV/dT markers are shown as short vertical white lines on each unipolar electrogram.

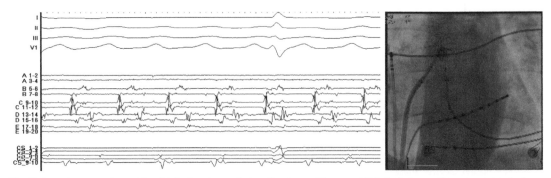

Fig. 5. Invasive mapping with a high-density catheter (Pentaray, Biosense Webster) shows the presence of a large part of the AT cycle length of 226 milliseconds localized in the roof.

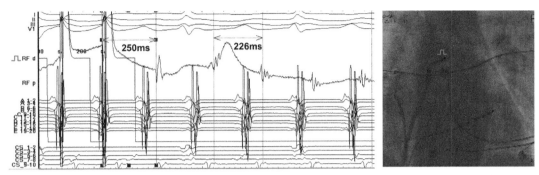

Fig. 6. Entrainment of AT shown in **Fig. 5** from the roof yielded post pacing interval 24 ms longer than the AT cycle length of 226 ms. The pacing rate was 200 ms.

the start of the third ablation procedure (**Fig. 3**). The perprocedural noninvasive map is shown in **Fig. 4**. Invasive mapping with the high-density catheter revealed the presence of a large part of the AT cycle length in the roof (**Fig. 5**). Entrainment from the roof yielded a postpacing interval (PPI) 24 milliseconds longer than the AT cycle length (**Fig. 6**). The PPI was much longer elsewhere in the left and right atrium (not shown). Ablation in the roof prolonged the tachycardia cycle length gradually until the AT converted to a slower focal source AT from the left atrium (not shown).

Clinical Case 3

A 72-year-old man underwent repeat ablation of persistent AF (6 months) refractory to 2 attempts of cardioversion assisted by antiarrhythmic drugs. The initial ablation procedure consisted of pulmonary vein isolation and cavotricuspid isthmus ablation. During ablation, AF converted to AT, which was consistent with counterclockwise perimitral AT on invasive mapping. Perprocedural noninvasive mapping revealed an activation pattern consistent with counterclockwise perimitral AT (**Fig. 7**). Ablation of the left mitral isthmus

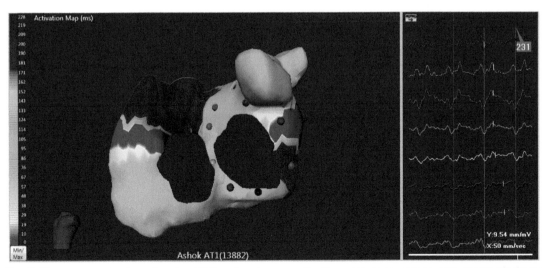

Fig. 7. The perprocedural noninvasive ECMap showing an activation pattern consistent with counterclockwise perimitral AT in a 72-year-old man undergoing repeat ablation of persistent AF of 6 months duration refractory to 2 attempts of cardioversion assisted by antiarrhythmic drugs. The color-coded time scale is seen on the left and the local unipolar electrograms during more than 3 AT cycles are displayed on the right. The color of the electrogram corresponds to the site of the same colored spot on the biatrial geometry. The –dV/dT markers are shown as short vertical white lines on each unipolar electrogram.

LAO View   PA View

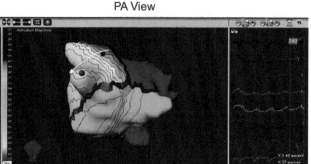

Fig. 8. Ablation of the left mitral isthmus converted counterclockwise perimitral AT shown in **Fig. 7** to double-loop AT (clockwise perimitral and roof-dependent circuits). The left panel shows an isochronal ECMap consistent with clockwise perimitral AT coexisting with a roof-dependent circuit shown in the isochronal ECMap in the right panel. The unipolar electrograms and their local activaton times ($-dV/dT$) are shown on the extreme right of the figure. The arrows show the direction of propagation of the wavefront.

converted counterclockwise perimitral AT to double-loop AT (clockwise perimitral [left panel of **Fig. 8**] and roof-dependent [right panel of **Fig. 8**] ATs), which was successfully ablated at the mitral isthmus followed by left atrial roof to sinus rhythm.

SUMMARY

Our experience with a novel, noninvasive, mapping system in a wide range of patients with and without previous ablation demonstrates the feasibility of accurately identifying the atria where AT is located and defining the AT mechanism. Recently developed algorithms based on regional and global atrial activation patterns combined with tissue level information such as local electrogram morphology and voltage have successfully helped overcome previous diagnostic limitations and improved the usefulness of the system in the noninvasive diagnosis of even the most complex forms of clinical ATs.

REFERENCES

1. Shah AJ, Hocini M, Xhaet O, et al. Validation of novel 3D electrocardiographic mapping of atrial tachycardias by invasive mapping and ablation: A multicenter study. J Am Coll Cardiol, in press.
2. Oster HS, Taccardi B, Lux RL, et al. Noninvasive electrocardiographic imaging: reconstruction of epicardial potentials, electrograms, and isochrones and localization of single and multiple electrocardiac events. Circulation 1997;96:1012–24.
3. Ramanathan C, Ghanem RN, Jia P, et al. Noninvasive electrocardiographic imaging for cardiac electrophysiology and arrhythmia. Nat Med 2004;10:422–8.
4. Rudy Y, Burnes JE. Noninvasive electrocardiographic imaging. Ann Noninvasive Electrocardiol 1999;4:340–58.
5. Saoudi N, Cosio F, Waldo A, et al. Classification of atrial flutter and regular atrial tachycardia according to electrophysiologic mechanism and anatomic bases: a statement from a joint expert group from the Working Group of Arrhythmias of the European Society of Cardiology and the North American Society of Pacing and Electrophysiology. J Cardiovasc Electrophysiol 2001;12(7):852–66.
6. Sanders P, Hocini M, Jaïs P, et al. Characterization of focal atrial tachycardia using high-density mapping. J Am Coll Cardiol 2005;46(11):2088–99.
7. Ghanem RN, Jia P, Ramanathan C, et al. Noninvasive electrocardiographic imaging (ECGI): comparison to intraoperative mapping in patients. Heart Rhythm 2005;2(4):339–54.
8. Intini A, Goldstein RN, Jia P, et al. Electrocardiographic imaging (ECGI), a novel diagnostic modality used for mapping of focal left ventricular tachycardia in a young athlete. Heart Rhythm 2005; 2(11):1250–2.

Index

Note: Page numbers of article titles are in **boldface** type.

Printed and bound by CPI Group (UK) Ltd, Croydon, CR0 4YY

03/10/2024

01040346-0011